DR. BACH'S FLOWER ESSENCES...

A QUANTUM APPROACH TO PRESCRIBING

ESMERALDA FUCCI, N.D., PH.D.

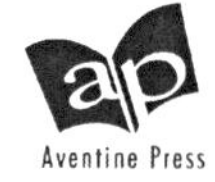

Aventine Press

Copyright© 2008 by Esmeralda A. Fucci
Cover Copyright© 2010 by Esmeralda A. Fucci

Without limiting the rights under copyright reserved above, no part of this publication may be reproduced, stored in or introduced into a retrieval system, or transmitted, in any form or by any means (electronic, mechanical, photocopying, recording, or otherwise), without the prior written permission of both the copyright owner and the publisher of this book.

Published by Aventine Press
750 State St. #319
San Diego CA, 92101
www.aventinepress.com

ISBN: 1-59330-645-8

Printed in the United States of America

ALL RIGHTS RESERVED

ACKNOWLEDGEMENT

My deepest gratitude to all the Great Ones: Dr. Hahnemann, Dr. Bach, et al., for their unsurpassed courage in discovering and utilizing healing systems that were in agreement with the highest healing principles of Nature, even when they went against the will of their allopathic counterparts; to my husband Ralph Luna, for his unconditional support and faith in my chosen profession and to my clients, whose health challenges and extraordinary trust placed in me, guided me to discovered new ways to facilitate their healing.

TABLE OF CONTENT

TABLE OF CONTENT   v

II.   FOREWORD   vii

III.   PREFACE   xi

IV.   INTRODUCTION   1

V.   BIOGRAPHY   7

VI.   DR. BACH'S HEALING SYSTEM   13

VII. DISEASE…ITS CAUSES AND CURE   19

VIII. REMEDY PREPARATION,
DOSAGE AND FREQUENCY   29

IX.   DR. BACH'S CLINICAL CASES   35

X.   RADIESTHESIA   41

XI.   CHRONINC DISEASES/MIASMS   47

XII. PROTOCOLS   67

XIII. AUTHOR'S CLINICAL CASES: 71
A) ANTI-MIASMATIC PROTOCOLS   73
B) MISCELLANEOUS PROTOCOLS   91

XIV. DR.BACH'S FLOWER ESSENCES
VIBRATIONAL CODES   113

XV. CLOSING STATEMENT   119

BIBLIOGRAPHY   123

FOREWORD

"Bacteria may play a role in disease but there are other factors outside the physical domain that render us or protect us against a disease."
Dr. Bach

FOREWORD

Dr. Edward Bach, in his address to the International Homeopathic Congress of 1927, honoring Dr. Samuel Hahnemann's contributions to the field of chronic toxaemia, stated:

"If I believe that I can make its nature clearer than was possible for him, I take no jot from his glory- rather I believe I am confirming and extending his work, and so paying him the only homage he would desire." *1

I trust that this book *confirms and extends* Dr. Edward Bach's work knowing that it would be *the only homage he would desire.*

*1. Bach, Dr., Edward, *The Problem of Chronic Disease*, International Homeopathic Congress, 1927; from the book: *Collected Writings of Edward Bach* (Ashgrove Publishing, England, 1987), p.204

PREFACE

" What we know as disease is the terminal stage of a much deeper disorder." Dr. Edward Bach

PREFACE

It has come to my attention via a variety of venues throughout my professional career, that Dr.Bach's Flower Essences were not effective in dealing with contemporary illnesses.

In order to ascertain the veracity of the above criticism I decided to research in depth Dr. Bach's healing system .The research journey that I embarked upon covered all of his surviving original writings and major publications of his system. Numerous other publications of various energy based healing systems, vibrational/energy medicine, Homeopathy,etc., written by North and South American, Indian and European scholars were also consulted. The outcome of this research, supported by the extensive clinical experience of the researcher, disputes the above stated criticism.

Furthermore, this research discovered a scientist with a profound respect for God's Creation and his fellow human beings. A person who made innumerable sacrifices in order to mitigate, if not cure, suffering and disease. An allopathic practitioner who was not afraid of loosing his medical license for the good of humanity when threaten on many occasions by the allopathic establishment. A person who honored and respected those who came before him and made discoveries that challenged the conventional thinking. An individual whose wholesomeness allowed him to maintain the child-like simplicity that rendered him access to unseen truths in order to achieve his high goals for the benefit of mankind. With the aid of Radiesthesia, Dr. Bach's flower essences have become indispensable in facilitating the healing process of my clients.

INTRODUCTION

" Nothing in nature can hurt us when we are happy and in harmony." Dr. Edward Bach

INTRODUCTION

If Dr. Edward Bach would be with us today, he would be considered an Energy Medicine Practitioner, or a Unified Field Medicine Practitioner. He was keenly aware of the unseen domain and its effect on the physical world. In the early part of the 20th century he often reminded us via his writings of the unity of all that has been created, seen and unseen. Dr. Bach knew, that the totality of Creation works in unity and harmony; that even a single thought can bring about imbalances. He repeatedly reminded us of being mindful of this concept of unity.

The unseen affects the seen. Science estimates that we are able to see 4% of what exists. However, those that are intuitive and sensitive to subtle energies operate with a much more expanded level of consciousness and a wider range of options to detect the unseen 96%.

Dr. Bach was a highly intuitive human being with a great understanding of materialistic science and a unique perception of the unseen forces affecting the physical domain and their role in curing diseases. His ultimate scientific and personal goal was to find a new system of healing that was simple and accessible to everyone and easy to learn and apply. He found this system later in his life and it had the *power to heal all types of illness and suffering.**1

According to Dr. Bach, *the disharmony between soul and mind* (*2) is the cause of disease. This conflict creates the stage of disease because it upsets the harmonious terrain that Creation depends on to properly function.

We live chaotic lives, our thoughts and actions lack harmony. We have upset the natural order with the resulting effect of suffering and disease. Dr. Bach's Healing System provides a way to harmonize disease causing energies thus opening up the channels for the mind and body to use its natural correcting and repairing mechanism to achieve lasting health. By removing these obstacles the body and mind heal themselves. This is accomplished, according to him, by these simplest of remedies that *have the power to elevate vibrations, and then draw down spiritual power, which cleanses mind and body, and heals. *3*

Via this remarkable insight he was led to design a system of healing that was both a mean to address this conflict and a system of cure that was to be both, easy to use and affordable by the general population.

During the period of research and development of his system of healing he was confronted with cases that did not fit the perimeters of standardization he was able to put together for the purpose of making it easy to use by the general population. Via his intuitive knowledge he was able to achieve good results by compensatory methods.

Today, when we are confronted with contemporary diseases/ imbalances, we find these to be too numerous and flower essences practitioners tend to neglect Dr.Bach's system seeking others that are marketed as being more relevant to these cases.

This phenomenon has created a trend of thought and belief that Dr. Bach's system is outdated, that our imbalances are too complex and fall outside of the energy range of his flower essences. The author of this book found this assertion incorrect.

It is true that the vibrational imbalances that exist today are quantifiably more complex than those that existed during his time. However, it is not true that these essences are not able to cure these imbalances. Quite to the contrary, they continue to be true healing herbs. They can still effectively address them. What is needed to make their application more successful is the adoption of an identification method more relevant to these contemporary imbalances. One that would be able to match the degree of these imbalances with the respective flower essence.

Clinical experience shows that in order to successfully deal with these cases, it is necessary to move beyond the traditional methods of diagnosis, remedy identification and dispensation. Crucial to achieve this goal is the adoption of an energy based method such as radiesthesia, that would be able to identify and quantify the imbalances at the energy level and match them with the proper flower essence.

This quantum approach makes Dr. Bach's Healing System as relevant today as it was during his time and it is also capable of detecting imbalances before they materialize on the physical, mental or emotional plane, such as non-manifested miasmatic tendencies.

In order to facilitate the understanding and dimension of Dr. Bach's contributions and their relevance to contemporary imbalances this book is organized as follows:

- A brief biography of Dr. Edward Bach
- A description of his healing system
- His concept of disease
- His way of preparing remedies, determining dosage and frequency
- An outline of his clinical records
- A brief overview of Dr. Hanemann's theory of chronic diseases/miasms
- A Radiesthesia narrative as the author's chosen energy based method
- A brief sample of the author's own clinical experience in treating chronic as well as acute conditions via the exclusive use of Dr. Bach's flower essences.

*1. Bach, Edward, Dr., *The Twelve Healers and Other Remedies*, 1936 (C.W.Daniel Co., England), page 4

*2. Bach, Edward, Dr., *Free Thyself, 1932; from The Original Writings of Edward Bach,* 1990 (St. Edmundsbury Press, England), page 50

*3. Bach, Edward, Dr., *Some Fundamental Considerations of Disease and Cure, Homeopathic World,* 1930, from the *Collected Writings of Edward Bach,* (Ashgrove Publishing, England), 1999, page 160

BIOGRAPHY

" Disease will never be cured or eradicated by present materialistic methods, for the simple reason that disease in its origin is not material."
Dr. Edward Bach

BIOGRAPHY

Dr. Edward Bach was born in Moseley, England on September 24, 1886.Since early childhood he demonstrated a high degree of sensitivity, compassion, a strong sense of purpose and a highly intuitive mind. His wish was to become an instrument of healing. These characteristics shepherded him to the world of science that culminated later in his life with the discovery of a unique system of healing.

He studied at Birmingham University and later on he went to London's University College Hospital where he finished his medical training in 1912. He became a homeopath, a pathologist and a bacteriologist.

As a medical student he did not allowed himself to be limited by the official medical textbook knowledge because he believed it was not the best source to facilitate healing. Instead he concentrated in observing the individual reactions of his patients and found out that their reactions to the same diseases were very different. Based upon this crucial observation he discovered that the same treatment did not cure the same disease.

He also noticed that individuals with similar personalities responded the same way to a specific remedy. Thus early in his career he concluded that the patient's personality was more important than the body in the treatment of a disease. He was very aware that he had to do a great deal of unlearning from medical school in order to be able to find a system of healing that was simple, universal and effective.

It made sense to him Dr. Hahnemann's approach of treating the patient rather than the disease; concentrating in identifying the cause of a disease rather than treating its symptoms. He also shared with him the belief that the physician's only mission is to cure those who are sick.

He discovered that poisoning from certain organisms in the intestines were the cause of chronic diseases. He prepared vaccines from these intestinal bacteria that were used successfully in the treatment of these chronic conditions. This method of treatment was widely adopted by the allopathic medical profession.

These vaccines were later developed as oral vaccines or nosodes. Dr. Bach had a profound dislike for any healing system or method that may cause pain. He believed that healing should be gentle, painless and benign.

He was then able to determine that the seven bacterial groups from which he made the vaccines corresponded to seven different personalities. Thus treating patients according to their personality symptoms with the appropriate nosodes he was able to achieve excellent healing results. However these nosodes represented only one type of diseases, the ones described by Dr. Hahnemann under the name of Psora, and did not cure all chronic diseases.

He then decided to research a purer system of healing that lead him to abandon, in 1930, his successful practice in London for a study of nature in the pursuit of this goal.

In 1928 he found the first of the 38 herbal remedies: Impatiens, Mimulus and Clematis. The 38 remedies where to heal any disease and healing was achieved by treating the patient's temperament/moods, not the disease.

In his search for a natural healing system he was faced with the issue of polarity. He found that nature's herbal remedies when potentized were of a positive polarity and those that were associated with disease were of a negative polarity, which were essential to achieve the results of bacterial nosodes.

Two years later he discovered a new form of potentization that removed the issue of polarity. He knew that he was on the right path to find a new system of healing.

From London he went to Wales. He believed that the plants with the proper medical properties were to be found among the simple wild flowers of the countryside. In Abersoch he perfected the sun method of extracting the medicinal properties of wild plants and wrote the book Heal Thyself. In this book he concludes that disease is the product of a conflict between the personality and the soul. By removing this conflict the disease will disappear.

Mimulus, Clematis, Impatiens, Agrimony, Chicory, Vervain, Centaury, Cerato and Scleranthus were the first nine remedies. By January of 1933 he found the first 12 remedies that corresponded to the twelve personality types. He wrote the book The Twelve Healers.

The next remedies will deal with states of mind more severe than the first twelve. He found Gorse, Oak, Heather and Rock Water. He named them The Four Helpers. He wrote the book The Twelve Healers and Four Helpers. Later he discovered Wild Oat, Olive and Vine. On July 1934 he published The Twelve Healers and Seven Helpers.

During the winter of 1933 and early spring of 1934 he was in Cromer treating patients. Here he prepared the Rescue Remedy. He was becoming more intuitive and powerful in his healings.

The second 19 remedies were found in a very different set of circumstances. For some days before the discovery of each one he suffered from the state of mind for which that particular remedy was required. The first of these remedies was Cherry Plum in March of 1935. During the following six months the other 18 remedies were found. On August of 1935 he potentized the last remedy. On September of 1936 the book the Twelve Healers and Other Remedies was published.

Dr. Bach felt that the best way to make the public aware of this new system of healing was via a lecture tour. The first lecture he gave it himself in Wallingford on the day of his fiftieth birthday, September 24, 1936. Towards the end of October his health begun to fail and on November 27, 1936 he died in his sleep. Shortly before his passing he destroyed all records of his work that he deemed irrelevant or that could lead to misinterpretation of his new system of healing.

From 1930 to 1936 he only used the herbal remedies for the treatment of all diseases.

DR. BACH'S HEALING SYSTEM

"These are the real causes of disease: restraint, fear, restlessness, indecision, indifference, weakness, doubt, over-enthusiasm, ignorance, impatience, terror and grief." Dr. Edward Bach

DR. BACH'S HEALING SYSTEM

In the introduction to the last edition of *The Twelve Healers and Other Remedies*, Dr. Bach summarizes the hallmark of his healing system:
- It is the most perfect healing system. *1
- It has the power to cure all types of illness and suffering. *2
- It is very simple to use. *3
- It is our fears, cares, anxieties, etc. that open the path to illness. *4
- Its remedies have proved that they are blest above others and that they have been given the power to heal all types of illness and suffering.*5
- In this healing system no notice is given to the nature of the disease. Only the mood of the patient is taken into account. *6
- As the individual mood is treated and the patient becomes well the disease goes, having been cast off by the increase of health. *7
- This healing system comprises 38 remedies that address 38 different moods or states of mind. *8

In an article published in the Homeopathic World, 1930, entitled *Some Fundamental Considerations of Disease and Cure*, Dr. Bach states:
"Another great principle of Hahnemann's genius may be considered here: the teaching of curing from within out. The mind must be healed first and the body will follow. To cure the body and not the mind might be very serious for the patient, as the body gains at the expense of the soul and at best it is a lesson deferred." *9

The above excerpt clearly illustrates why Dr. Bach considered his work to be a continuation of that of Dr. Hahnemann's and why his system of healing centers around the moods of the patient.

A crucial premise of his scientific discovery was his belief that disease is the result of a conflict between the personality (mind) and the soul. By aligning the personality with the soul, disease will disappear. The 38 remedies of this system of healing addresses all of the negative moods.

Dr. Bach honored those who passed before him and made a positive contribution to humanity. In his 1931 lecture *Ye Suffer From Yourselves*, he mentioned that:

" Hanemann, like Paracelsus, knew that if our spiritual and mental aspects were in harmony, illness could not exist. So in his new system of healing the mind state is of paramount importance." *10

In his book *Heal Thyself*, Dr. Bach explains why the mind is central to this system of healing:

" The mind being the most delicate and sensitive part of the body, shows the onset and the course of disease much more definitely than the body, so that the outlook of the mind is chosen as the guide as to which remedy or remedies are necessary. Take no notice of the disease, think only of the outlook on life of the one in distress." *11

How these remedies work is explained in different ways but with a common element: these remedies were of the highest energy/ vibration rate.

In an article published in the Homeopathic World in 1930, entitled *Some Fundamental Considerations of Disease and Cure*, Dr. Bach wrote:

" It is essential that remedies chosen should be life-giving and uplifting; of such vibrations that elevate… and thus draw down the spiritual power, which cleanses mind and body, and heals." *12

In his lecture entitled: *Ye Suffer From Yourselves*, he said:

" These remedies, which have been Divinely enriched with healing powers, will be administered to open up those channels to allow more of the light of the Soul, that the patient may be flooded with healing virtue…The action of these remedies is to raise our vibrations and open up the channels for the reception of our spiritual self, to flood our natures with the particular virtue we need and wash out from us the fault which is causing harm…They cure not by attacking the disease but by flooding our bodies with the beautiful vibrations of our Higher Nature, in the presence of which disease melts as snow in the sunshine." *13

In a 1935 letter to a colleague, he writes:

" There is no doubt that these new remedies act on a different plane to the old. They are more spiritualized and help us to develop that inner great self in all of us which has the power to overcome all fears, all worries ALL diseases." *14

In a letter written on October 26, 1936, a month before his passing, he wrote:

" There has been disclosed unto us a system of healing such as has not been known within the memory of men; when, with the simplicity of the herbal remedies, we can set forth with the certainty, the absolute certainty, of their power to conquer disease." *15

Furthermore, these remedies have the power to preserve the positive qualities of our personalities, thus achieving harmony with our higher self.

In his book *Heal Thyself*, he states:

" The remedies assist us to maintain our personality… The remedies will help the physical body to gain strength, to assert the mind to become calm, widen the outlook and strive towards perfection, thus bringing peace and harmony to the whole personality." *16

In his book *Free Thyself* he writes: " All we have to do is preserve our personality. The healing herbs are those which have been given the power to help us preserve our personality." *17

*1.   Bach, Edward, *The Twelve Healers and Other Remedies,* 1936 (Vermilion Publishing, England, 2005), page 3

*2.   Bach, Edward, *The Twelve Healers and Other Remedies,* 1936 (Vermilion Publishing, England, 2005), page 4

*3.   Bach, Edward, *The Twelve Healers and Other Remedies,* 1936 (Vermilion Publishing, England, 2005), page 3

*4.   Bach, Edward, *The Twelve Healers and Other Remedies,* 1936 (Vermilion Publishing, England, 2005), page 3

*5.   Bach, Edward, *The Twelve Healers and Other Remedies,* 1936 (Vermilion Publishing, England, 2005), page 4

*6.   Bach, Edward, *The Twelve Healers and Other Remedies,* 1936 (Vermilion Publishing, England, 2005) page 4

*7.   Bach, Edward, *The Twelve Healers and Other Remedies,* 1936 (Vermilion Publishing, England, 2005), page 4

*8.   Bach, Edward, *The Twelve Healers and Other Remedies,* 1936 (Vermilion Publishing, England, 2005) page 5

*9.   Bach, Edward, *Some Fundamental Considerations of Disease and Cure,* 1930, Homeopathic World; from *Collected Writings of Edward Bach* (Ashgrove Publishing, England, 1999), page 160

*10.   Bach, Edward, *Ye Suffer From Yourselves,* 1931; from *Collected Writings of Edward Bach,* (Ashgrove Publishing, England, 1999) page 111

*11.   Bach, Edward, *Heal Thyself,* 1931 (C.W. Daniel, England, 1996), Foreword, page 2

*12.   Bach, Edward, *Some fundamental Considerations of Disease and Cure,* 1930, Homeopathic World; from *Collected Writings of Edward Bach* (Ashgrove Publishing, England, 1999), page 160

*13.   Bach, Edward, *Ye suffer From Yourselves,* 1931; from *Collected Writings of Edward Bach* (Ashgrove Publishing, England, 1999), page 117

*14.   Bach, Edward, July 1, 1935 letter to a colleague, from *Collected Writings of Edward Bach* (Ashgrove Publishing, England, 1999), page 23

*15.   Bach, Edward, October 26, 1936 letter from *Collected Writings of Edward Bach* (Ashgrove Publishing, England, 1999), page 32

*16.   Bach, Edward, *Heal Thyself,* 1931 (C.W. Daniel Company Limited, 1996), page 40

*17.   Bach, Edward, *Free Thyself,* 1932; from *Collected Writings of Edward Bach* (Ashgrove Publishing, England, 1999), page 95

DISEASE
ITS CAUSES AND CURE

" Suffering is corrective to point out a lesson which by other means we have failed to grasp and never can it be eradicated until that lesson is learnt." Dr. Edward Bach

DISEASE…ITS CAUSES AND CURE

DISEASE CAUSE

Dr. Edward Bach considered disease a symptom of a more severe condition. He made a distinction between affections caused by bacteria, accidents, poisons, etc. and diseases due to a more serious cause. In his book Heal Thyself he says:

" Bacteria may play a role in disease but there are other factors outside the physical domain that render us or protect us against a disease." *1

" Certain maladies may be caused by direct physical means, such as those associated with poisons, accidents, etc; but disease in general is due to some basic error in our constitution. Thus a complete cure requires a physical mean and also the removal of any fault in our nature because final and complete healing ultimately comes from within, from the soul itself, which radiates harmony throughout the personality, when allow to do so." *2

" What we know as disease is the terminal stage of a much deeper disorder." *3

" Disease will never be cured or eradicated by present materialistic methods for the simple reason that disease in its origin is not material. What we know as disease is an ultimate result produce in the body, the end product of deep and long acting forces." *4

In his 1931 article Ye Suffer From Yourselves he states:

" Disease of the body, as we know it, is the result and end product, a final stage of something much deeper. It originates above the physical plane, nearer to the mental." *5

He places the origin of disease at the schism point between the personality and the Soul. In his 1931 lecture Ye Suffer from Yourselves he states that disease is:

" Entirely the result of a conflict between our spiritual and mortal selves. So long as these two are in harmony, we are in perfect health; but when there is discord, there follows what we know as disease." *6

In Free Thyself he says:

" Disease of the body itself is nothing but the result of the disharmony between the soul and the mind. It is only a symptom of the cause and as the same cause will manifest itself differently in nearly every individual, seek to remove this cause." *7

In his book Heal Thyself repeatedly he stresses this point:

" Disease is in essence the result of conflict between Soul and mind and will never be eradicated except by spiritual and mental effort." *8

" Conflict between Soul and personality is the primary basic cause of disease." *9

" Every Soul is here for the specific purpose of gaining experience and understanding and of perfecting his personality towards these ideals laid down by the Soul. Unless this work is done, a conflict between his Soul and personality will arise, which of necessity will react in forms of physical disorders." *10

" So long as our personalities are in harmony all is joy and peace, happiness and health. It is when our personalities are led from the path laid down by the soul, either by our own worldly desires or by the persuasion of others, that a conflict arises. This conflict is the root cause of disease and unhappiness." *11

" Our outlook in life depends on the nearness of the personality to the soul. The closer the union the greater the harmony and peace." *12

" There are two great errors:

(1) Dissociation between our Souls and our personality.

(2) Cruelty or wrong to others, for this is a sin against unity. Either of these brings conflict, which leads to disease." *13

The conflict between the personality/mind and the Soul is manifested in different ways. In his 1932 book Free Thyself he states:

" These are the real causes of disease: Restraint, fear, restlessness, indecision, indifference, weakness, doubt, over-enthusiasm, ignorance, impatience, terror, grief." *14

THE BENEFITIAL ROLE OF DISEASE

Dr. Bach believed that disease has a useful and redeeming role. In his 1931 lecture Ye Suffer From Yourselves he says:

" Disease is solely and purely corrective: It is neither vindictive nor cruel. But it is the means adopted by our own Soul to point to us our faults, to prevent our making greater errors, to hinder us from doing more harm and to bring us back to that path of truth and light from which we should never have strayed. Disease is in reality for our good, and is beneficient, though we should avoid it if we had but the correct understanding, combined with the desire to do right. " *15

In his book Heal Thyself he writes:

" Let it briefly state that disease, tough apparently so cruel, is in itself beneficient and for our good and if rightly interpreted it will guide us to our essential faults. If properly treated it will be the cause of the removal of those faults and leave us better and greater than before… Suffering is corrective to point out a lesson which by other means we have failed to grasp and never can it be eradicated until that lesson is learnt." *16

" Any type of illness from which we may suffer will guide us to the discovery of the fault which lies behind our afflictions." *17

" Disease is in itself beneficient and has for its object the bringing back of the personality to the Divine will of the Soul." *18

HOW TO CONQUER DISEASE

In his book Heal Thyself Dr. Bach states that in order to conquer disease the following must take place:

1. "Realize the divinity within yourself and the power we have to overcome all that is wrong.
2. Know that the cause of disease is due to disharmony between the personality and the soul.
3. Be willing to discover the fault that is causing such a conflict.
4. Remove such a fault by developing the opposite virtue." *19

He strongly believed that these steps would prevent illness because:

- " Bringing about harmony between body, mind and Soul will cure disease." *20

In Twelve Healers:
" There are seven steps in healing in the following order:
Peace, hope, joy, faith, certainty, wisdom, and love; and once love enters into the patient, not self-love, but the love of the universe, then he has turned his back on what we call disease." *21
In The Twelve Healers and Seven Helpers:
"There is no disease of itself which is incurable." *22
" In this age, in saying these herbs can cure all disease it is necessary to add: In those who really desire to get well, because under present conditions, illness often brings advantages to a patient which sometimes he does not truly desire to lose." *23
" It does not matter what the disease is, the mood alone has to be treated." *24
From the Masonic Lecture of October, 1936 we find:
" The message is this: That disease is Curable. By the means of the herbs of I am speaking tonight, there is no ordinary disease known in this country which has not been cured…So in healing with these herbs, the body is not taken into any account, whatever may be wrong with it is of no consideration. All we seek are those characters of the sufferer where he is in disharmony with the well of peace in his Soul…An by the treatment with Divine Herbs of Healing, these adverse qualities will disappear, so with their disappearance, no matter what the disease, the body becomes well."*25
In The Twelve Healers and Four Helpers:
"In this book is given the description of twelve herbs that have the power to cure all types of disease…" *26
In Free Thyself:
"In true healing there is no thought whatever of the disease: it is the mental state, the mental difficulty alone, to be considered: it is where we are wrong in the Divine Plan that matters." *27

In The Twelve Healers And Other Remedies he describes the 38 remedies and places them under seven headings. They are:

1- Fear: Rock Rose, Mimulus, Cherry Plum, Aspen, Red Chestnut.
2- Uncertainty: Cerato, Scleranthus, Gentian, Gorse, Hornbeam, Wild Oat.

3- Insufficient interest in present circumstances: Clematis, Honeysuckle, Wild Rose, Olive, White Chestnut, Mustard, Chestnut Bud.

4- Loneliness: Water Violet, Impatiens, Heather.

5- Over-sensitive to influences and ideas: Agrimony, Centaury, Walnut, Holly.

6- Despondency and despair: Larch, Elm, Sweet Chestnut, Star of Bethlehem, Willow, Oak, Crab Apple.

7- Over-care for the welfare of others: Chicory, Vervain, Vine, Beech, Rock Water." *28

" In treating cases with these remedies no notice is taken of the nature of the disease. The individual is treated and as he becomes well the disease goes, having been cast off by the increased health… Take no notice of the disease, think only of the outlook on life of the one in distress." *29

In Heal Thyself:

" Healing will pass from the domain of physical methods of treating the physical body to that of spiritual and mental healing, which, by bringing about harmony between the Soul and mind, will eradicate the very basic cause of disease." *30

Dr. Bach's flower essences represent a holistic system of healing. I addresses the needs of the body, mind and spirit; it offers guidelines for the maintenance of health and prevention of illnesses, and in cases of actual diseases, it provides the necessary remedies that will stimulate the healing process.

*1. Bach, Edward, Dr., *Heal Thyself*, 1931 (C.W. Daniel Co., England, 1996), p.48

*2. Bach, Edward, Dr., *Heal Thyself,* 1931 (C.W. Daniel Co., England, 1996), p.17

*3. Bach, Edward, Dr., *Heal Thyself*, 1931 (C.W. Daniel Co., England, 1996), p.11

*4. Bach, Edward, Dr., *Heal Thyself,* 1931 (C.W. Daniel Co., England, 1996), p.2

*5. Bach, Edward, Dr., *Ye Suffer From Yourselves*, 1931; from *Collected Writings of Edward Bach* (Asgrove Publishing, England, 1999), p.114

*6. Bach, Edward, Dr., *Ye Suffer From Yourselves*, 1931, from *Collected Writings of Edward Bach* (Ashgrove Publishing, England, 1999), p.114

*7. Bach, Edward, Dr., *Free Thyself,* 1932, from *Collected Writings of Edward Bach* (Ashgrove Publishing, England, 1999), pp.100 and 101

*8. Bach, Edward, Dr., *Heal Thyself,* 1931 (C.W. Daniel Co., England, 1996), p.2

*9. Bach, Edward, Dr., *Heal Thyself,* 1931 (C.W. Daniel Co., England, 1996), p.24

*10. Bach, Edward, Dr., *Heal Thyself,* 1931 (C.W. Daniel Co., England, 1996), p.30

*11. Bach, Edward, Dr., *Heal Thyself,* 1931 (C.W. Daniel Co., England, 1996), p.7

*12. Bach, Edward, Dr., *Heal Thyself,* 1931 (C.W. Daniel Co., England, 1996), p.55

*13. Bach, Edward, Dr., *Heal Thyself,* 1931 (C.W. Daniel Co., England, 1996), p.8

*14. Bach, Edward, Dr., *Free Thyself,* 1932, from *Collected Writings of Edward Bach* (Ashgrove Publishing, England, 1999), p.14

*15. Bach, Edward, Dr., *Ye Suffer From Yourselves*, 1931; from *Collected Writings of Edward Bach* (Ashgrove Publishing, England, 1999), p.114

*16.   Bach, Edward, Dr., *Heal Thyself,* 1931 (C.W. Daniel Co., England, 1996), p.4

*17. Bach, Edward, Dr., *Heal Thyself,* 1931 (C.W. Daniel Co., England, 1996), p.14

*18. Bach, Edward, Dr., *Heal Thyself,* 1931 (C.W. Daniel Co., England, 1996), p. 9

*19. Bach, Edward, Dr., *Heal Thyself,* 1931 (C.W. Daniel Co., England, 1996), p. 52

*20. Bach, Edward, Dr., *Heal Thyself,* 1931 (C.W. Daniel Co., England, 1996), p.53

*21. Bach, Edward, Dr., *Twelve Healers*, 1933, from *Collected Writings of Edward Bach* (Ashgrove Publishing, England, 1999), p.79

*22. Bach, Edward, Dr., *The Twelve Healers and Seven Helpers*, 1934 (C.W. Daniel Co., England), p.51

*23. Bach, Edward, Dr., *The Twelve Healers and Seven Helpers*, 1934 (C.W. Daniel Co., England), pp. 56 and 57

*24. Bach, Edward, Dr., *The Twelve Healers and Seven Helpers*, 1934 (C.W. Daniel Co., England), p.52

*25. Bach, Edward, Dr., Ma*sonic Lecture of October, 1936*, from *Collected Writings of Edward Bach* (Ashgrove Publishing, England, 1999), p.11

*26. Bach, Edward, Dr., *The Twelve Healers and Four Helpers*, 1933 (C.W. Daniel Co., England), p.1

*27. Bach, Edward, Dr., *Free Thyself, 1932*; from *Collected Writings of Edward Bach* (Ashgrove Publishing, England, 1999), p. 103

*28. Bach, Edward, Dr., *The Twelve Healers and Other Remedies*, 1931 (Vermilion Publishing, 2005), pp. 5-24

*29. Bach, Edward, Dr., *The Twelve Healers and Other Remedies*, 1931 (Vermilion Publishing, England, 2005), p.4

*30. Bach, Edward, Dr., *Heal Thyself*, 1931 (C.W. Daniel Co., England, 1996), p.39

REMEDY PREPARATION, DOSAGE AND FREQUENCY

" There are seven steps in healing in the following order: Peace, Hope, Joy, Faith, Certainty, Wisdom, and Love." Dr. Edward Bach

REMEDY PREPARATION, DOSAGE AND FREQUENCY

Dr. Bach administered the flower essences intuitively. He was able to "know" how much the patient needed. In his quest to develop a system of healing that would be easily understood by the public at large, attempts were made to establish guidelines with regards to remedy preparation, dosage and frequency of remedy delivery in different publications. The following are some of these guidelines.

REMEDY PREPARATION AND DOSAGE:
" Take an ordinary four-ounce medicine bottle, pour into this 4 drops from the stock bottle of the required remedy, fill-up with water and shake well. This is the medicine which is given to the patient in doses of a teaspoonful as necessary". *1

" One drop alone of this is sufficient to make potent an eight ounce bottle of water from which doses may be taken by the tea-spoonful as required". *2

" The dosage is as follows: take two or three drops of the stock remedy to an ordinary medicine bottle, fill it with water, shake up well, then give teaspoonfuls of this as required". *3

" Take a cupful of water and add only 3 or four drops from the little bottles supplied by the chemist of the needful herb or herbs, and stir it up. To children give an egg- spoonful, and for grown-ups a teaspoonful at a time". *4

" Two drops from the stock bottle with a small bottle nearly filled with water: if this is required to keep for some time, a little brandy may be added as a preservative. The bottle is used for giving doses, and but a few drops of this, taken in a little water, milk, or any way convenient, is all that it is necessary". *5

DOSE FREQUENCY:

" In very urgent cases doses may be given quite often, as frequently as every quarter of an hour. If the patient is unconscious it is sufficient merely to moisten the lips with the remedy. In serious cases where the patient has chronic complaint the rule to follow is to give a dose whenever the patient feels the need, whether this be eight or ten times a day or only once or twice." *6

" The doses should be taken as the patient feels it necessary: Hourly in acute cases; three or four time a day in chronic cases until relief occurs " *7

" In urgent cases every quarter of an hour, in serious cases every hour, and in ordinary cases three or four times daily." *8

" In very desperate cases doses may be given every quarter of an hour; in severe cases, every hour, and in ordinary long-standing illness about every two or three hours spread over the day or more often if the patient feels it is helping to take it frequently." *9

" In urgent cases the doses may be given every few minutes, until there is improvement; in severe cases about half-hourly; and in long standing cases every two or three hours or more often or less as the patient feels the need. In those unconscious, moisten lips frequently." *10

Remedies were delivered orally, or via a lotion or a compress. The length of treatment varied from a single dose to multiple doses; from one time treatment to months long treatments. All of them determined either intuitively or by the patient's determination that she/he needed more doses of the remedy. With regards to how many remedies could be used during the course of a given treatment, the records shows from 1 to up to 6 or up to 9.

" As the patient improves it will often be found necessary to change the remedy as his state changes, and in some cases as many as half a dozen different herbs may be required". *11

" The number of remedies chosen at any one time varies with the individual needs. For some only one or two were needed, for others five or six, and on some occasions eight or nine". *12

*1.   Bach, Edward, Dr., *The Twelve Healers and Four Helpers*, 1933, from *Collected Writings of Edward Bach* (Ashgrove Publishing, England, 1999), p.67

*2.   Bach, Edward, Dr., *Twelve Healers*, 1933, from *Collected Writings of Edward Bach* (Ashgrove Publishing, England, 1999), p.81

*3.   Bach, Edward, Dr., *Twelve Great Remedies*, 1933, from *Collected Writings of Edward Bach* (Ashgrove Publishing, 1999), p.83

*4.   Bach, Edward, Dr., *The Twelve Healers and Seven Helpers*, 1934, from *Collected Writings of Edward Bach* (Ashgrove Publishing, 1999), p.57

*5.   Bach, Edward, Dr., *The Twelve Healers and Other Remedies*, 1936, from *Collected Writings of Edward Bach* (Ashgrove, England, 1999), pp.46-47

*6.   Bach, Edward, Dr., *The* Twelve *Healers and Four Helpers*, 1933, from *Collected Writings of Edward Bach* (Ashgrove Publishing, England, 1999), p.67

*7.   Bach, Edward, Dr., *Twelve Healers*, 1933, from *Collected Writings of Edward Bach* (Ashgrove Publishing, 1999), p.81

*8.   Bach, Edward, Dr., *Twelve Great Remedies,* 1933, from *Collected Writings of Edward Bach* (Ashgrove Publishing, England, 1999), p.83

*9.   Bach, Edward, Dr., *The Twelve Healers and Seven Helpers*, 1934, from *Collected Writings of Edward Bach* (Ashgrove Publishing, 1999, England), p. 57

*10.   Bach, Edward, Dr., *The Twelve Healers and Other Remedies*, 1936, from *Collected Writings of Edward Bach* (Ashgrove Publishing, England, 1999),p.p. 46-47

*11.   Bach, Edward, Dr., *Twelve Great Remedies*, 1933, from *Collected Writings of Edward Bach* (Ashgrove Publishing, 1999), p.85

*12.   Howard, Judy and Ramsell, John, *The Original Writings of Edward Bach*, (C.W. Daniel Co., England, 1990), p.113

DR.BACH'S
CLINICAL CASES

"There is no disease of itself which is incurable" Dr. Edward Bach

DR.BACH'S CLINICAL CASES

CONDITION		CLIENT	FLOWER ESSENCE
ALCOHOLISM	*1	FEMALE (47 yrs. old)	AGRIMONY
ACCIDENT	*2	MALE	AGRIMONY
APATHY	*3	MALE (37 yrs. old)	CLEMATIS
ASTHMA	*4	MALE (8 yrs. old)	AGRIMONY
ASTHMA	*5	FEMALE (36 yrs. old)	CLEMATIS
ASTHMA	*6	FEMALE (30 yrs. old)	CLEMATIS, GORSE
ASTHMA	*7	FEMALE (40 yrs. old)	AGRIMONY
ASTHMA	*8	FEMALE (38 yrs. old)	CLEMATIS
BLEEDING	*9	FEMALE (9 yrs. old)	CENTAURY
CYST	*10	FEMALE (18 yrs. old)	CLEMATIS
DEAFNESS	*11	FEMALE (38 yrs. old)	CHICORY
DEPRESSION	*12	FEMALE	OAK, CLEMATIS ROCK ROSE
ELECTRO-CUTION	*13	MALE (21 yrs. old)	CLEMATIS, AGRIMONY, MIMULUS, ROCK ROSE, SCLERANTHUS, GENTIAN
HERNIA	*14	MALE (22yrs. old)	CERATO

INDIGESTION	*15	FEMALE	CHICORY
LEUKEMIA	*16	FEMALE (40 yrs. old)	ROCK ROSE, MIMULUS
MEMORY LOSS	*17	MALE (47 yrs. old)	CLEMATIS
NERVES	*18	MALE (55 yrs. old)	SCLERANTHUS
PARALYSIS	*19	MALE	VERVAIN
PAIN	*20	FEMALE (40 yrs. old)	ROCK ROSE, MIMULUS
PAIN	*21	FEMALE (22 yrs. old)	GORSE, CLEMATIS
PAIN	*22	MALE	SCLERANTHUS
RHEUMATISM	*23	FEMALE	WATER VIOLET, CHICORY, IMPATIENS, SCLERANTHUS
RHEUMATISM	*24	MALE (35 yrs. old)	AGRIMONY, MIMULUS, GENTIAN
RHEUMATISM	*25	MALE (64 yrs. old)	VERVAIN
RHEUMATISM	*26	MALE (38 yrs. old)	AGRIMONY MIMULUS GENTIAN
RHEUMATISM	*27	FEMALE	WATER VIOLET, IMPATIENS, SCLERANTHUS
SKIN RASH	*28	FEMALE	CERATO
SLEEP DISORDER	*29	FEMALE (40 yrs. old)	CLEMATIS
SPRAIN	*30	MALE (50 yrs. old)	IMPATIENS
SWELLING (GLANDS)	*31	MALE (8 yrs. old)	AGRIMONY, CHICORY, ROCK ROSE,

			CLEMATIS, CENTAURY, GENTIAN
TUBERCULAR *32 (HIP JOINTS)		FEMALE	AGRIMONY, IMPATIENS, GORSE, OAK
WART	*33	MALE (40 yrs. old)	HEATHER
WEAKNESS	*34	FEMALE (11 yrs. old)	CENTAURY

*1   The Medical Discoveries of Edward Bach, p.72   **1

*2   The Medical Discoveries of Edward Bach, p. 71

*3   The Original Writings of Edward Bach, p.119   **2

*4   The Medical Discoveries of Edward Bach,p.71

*5   The Medical Discoveries of Edward Bach, p.76

*6   The Medical Discoveries of Edward Bach, p.97

*7   The Medical Discoveries of Edward Bach, p.86

*8   The Medical Discoveries of Edward Bach, p.121

*9   The Medical Discoveries of Edward Bach, p.77

*10   Collected Writings of Edward Bach, p.85   **3

*11   The Medical Discoveries of Edward Bach, p.73

*12   The Medical Discoveries of Edward Bach, p.99

*13   The Original Writings of Edward Bach, p.122

*14   The Medical Discoveries of Edward Bach, p.77

*15   The Medical Discoveries of Edward Bach, p.73

*16   Collected Writings of Edward Bach, p.85

*17   The Original Writings of Edward Bach, p.120

*18   The Medical Discoveries of Edward Bach, p.79

*19   Collected Writings of Edward Bach, p.86

*20   Collected Writings of Edward Bach, p.85

*21   The Medical Discoveries of Edward Bach, p.98

*22   The Medical Discoveries of Edward Bach, p.75

*23   Collected Writings of Edward Bach, p.85

*24   Collected Writings of Edward Bach, p.85

*25   The Medical Discoveries of Edward Bach, p.74
*26   The Medical Discoveries of Edward Bach, p.92
*27   The Medical Discoveries of Edward Bach, p.92
*28   The Medical Discoveries of Edward Bach, p.76
*29   The Medical Discoveries of Edward Bach, p.78
*30   The Medical Discoveries of Edward Bach, p.74
*31   The Medical Discoveries of Edward Bach, p.91
*32   The Medical Discoveries of Edward Bach, p.99
*33   The Medical Discoveries of Edward Bach, p.98
*34   The Medical Discoveries of Edward Bach, p.78

**1   Weeks, Nora. "The Medical Discoveries of Dr. Bach, Physician",
        1973 New Canaan, Ct. Keats Publishing Company, England.
**2   Barnard, Julian, Editor. "Collected Writings of Edward Bach:,
        1987. Ashgrove Publishing, London, England.
**3   Howard, Judy and Ramsell, John. "The Original Writings of
        Edward Bach", 1990. The C.W. Daniel Company Limited,
        London, England.

RADIESTHESIA

" It does not matter what the disease is, the mood alone has to be treated." Dr. Edward Bach

RADIESTHESIA

Dr. Edward Bach, even with his extraordinary intuition, had problems identifying the correct remedies.

In his book The Twelve Healers and Four Helpers*1 he states:

" It will be found that certain cases do not seem to fit exactly any of the Twelve Healers…" *1

He resorted to different methods to correct these difficulties. In his book The Twelve Healers and Seven Helpers he says:

" If the patient does not improve when what seems the right one of the healers has been given, there are seven more remedies to prepare the way…which are called the seven helpers." *2

" Wild Oat may be required by anyone, and if what seems to be the right one of the Healers or the right one of the Helpers does not give benefit, in all such cases try the remedy Wild Oat." *3

" If a remedy that may be needed by anyone, and in cases which do not respond to herbs (meaning the flower essences.), or when it seems difficult to decide which to give, try this (Wild Oat) for at least a week." *4

Nowadays, it is more difficult to ascertain the right remedy and it is not because they are not relevant to contemporary imbalances/ diseases. The world is faced with a number of factors that have upset the natural balance. An example of this is electromagnetic pollution (EMF). Regarding EMF, Andrew Weil, M.D. states that it "may be the most significant form of pollution human activity has produced in this century, all the most dangerous because it is invisible and insensible". There is not a single second during our daily lives that we are not being exposed to it. This type of environment is unprecedented in the history of human kind.

With the advent of radio, and television broadcasting stations, cordless phones, cell phones, computers, etc., radio waves and microwaves density in our mist are millions of times higher than natural levels. This does not take into account the Extreme Low Frequency (ELF) fields produced by electrical appliances.

Study after studies show that these energy fields have the effect of disrupting the natural energy balance of our bodies and minds. It has been proven that EMF can trigger stress responses of such a magnitude that negatively affect the body's ability to heal, and exhaust the energy level thus producing energy depletion with its concomitant fatigue, etc.

Living organisms are electromagnetic instruments with unique vibrational frequencies and both, EMF and ELF, can adversely affect their energy balance being capable of causing heart disease, cancer, Alzheimer, Parkinson, depression, fatigue, etc.

Today's world requires strengthened mental, emotional, and physical health. Dr. Bach's flower essences can play a significant role in bringing about spiritual, mental and physical health. However, what is needed to make his system of healing more relevant is to utilize an energy base technique to assess the degree of imbalance of today's very complex energy imbalances.

Clinical experience demonstrates that Dr. Bach's healing essences have the vibrational qualities to heal diseases. An energy base method, such as radiesthesia, muscle testing (a cruder form of radiesthesia), etc. can be invaluable in matching the right essence or combination of essences with a particular illness/imbalance.

Radiesthesia would have been a great instrument to even Dr. Bach, particularly in those cases that he had difficulties with ascertaining the right remedy or when the right remedy was chosen but was not producing the desired result. Furthermore, the practice of radiesthesia has the added benefit of augmenting, and integrating in a more balanced way our intuition.

Radiesthesia allows the practitioner to detect and quantify the energies that affect the mental/ physical/ soul harmony and match them with the healing energy pattern of the right flower essence. An experienced radiesthetist will also be able to achieve a short cut to the traditional way of identifying the right healing essence.

Radiesthesia is the science and the art of perceiving the subtle energies present in creation. From the Latin "radius", for radiation and the Greek " aesthesis" for sensibilidad.The term radiesthesia was introduced in 1930 by the French priest Abate Alexis Bouly, in order to substitute the word of Greek etimology " rabdomancia" (Rhabdos= stick and Manteia= adivination or prophesy), because radiesthesia has more affinity with the name of a practical and rational science, whereas rabdomancia suggests a relationship with magical powers. *5

As a practical science, radiesthesia is capable of detecting and measuring the entire spectrum of radiations/ subtle energies emitted from the entire cosmos: minerals, vegetables, animals and human beings. It is very important to point out that we all have within us the natural radiesthetic ability, but since we have not used it, we lost the ability to perceive these subtle energies. However it can be relearned.

Rev. Ricardo Luis Gerula, a prominent radiesthesist, says that this learning can be achieved by:
- Studying the principles of this science
- Becoming proficient in the techniques
- Practicing the techniques.
- Developing an independent mental attitude, free of auto suggestions.
- Avoiding prejudices or preconceived ideas.
- Maintaining a personal conduct of prudence, modesty and discretion.
- Honoring professional confidentiality.
- Verifying the obtained results.
- Communicating and interpreting each finding as additional data to be taken into account with the overall findings.
- Remembering that nature rules itself by the principle of energy efficiency and it does not benefit itself when it has to utilize twice as much energy in achieving a single task. Thus if a data/ information can be obtained by a rational method, nature will not cooperate in producing this data/ information via an intuitive method such as radiesthesia.
- Being always very responsible and professional in the exercise of radiesthesia, a scientific method that can be very difficult to explain,

however, so unquestionable in its results. It is a bridging instrument between the seen (a material science domain) and the unseen (the quantum/ unifying field). *6

Radiesthesia is an excellent instrument for the identification and quantification of all physical or mental imbalances; selection of remedies, ways to formulate their dosage and order of dispensation, etc. It is particularly invaluable in cases that do not fit the traditional mode of identifying the right Bach's flower essences, which is very frequently the case with contemporary diseases. With it, the practitioner will be able to advance Bach's Healing System into the centuries beyond; a truly an indispensable instrument for a vibrational mode of healing.

*1.	Bach, Edward, Dr., *The Twelve Healers and Four Helpers*, 1933, from *Collected Writings of Edward Bach* (Ashgrove Publishing, England, 1999), p.69

*2.	Bach, Edward, Dr., *The Twelve Healers and Seven Helpers*, 1934, from *Collected Writings of Edward Bach* (Ashgrove Publishing, England, 1999), p.55

*3.	Bach, Edward, Dr., *The Twelve Healers and Seven Helpers*, 1934, from *Collected Writings of Edward Bach* (Ashgrove Publishing, England, 1999), p.55

*4.	Bach, Edward, Dr. *The Twelve Healers and Seven Helpers*, 1934, from *Collected Writings of Edward Bach* (Ashgrove Publishing, England, 1999), p.56

*5.	Gurula, Ricardo Luis, Reverend, *Radiestesia Integral, 2005* (Editorial Kier, Buenos Aires, Argentina, 2005), p.51

*6.	Gurula, Ricardo Luis, Reverend, *Radiestesia Integral, 2005* (Editorial Kier, Buenos Aires, Argentina, 2005), p.51

CHRONIC DISEASES/ MIASMS

" Health is our heritage. It is the complete and full union between soul, mind and body." Dr. Edward Bach

CHRONICC DISEASES/MIASMS

Searching for a place to practice medicine freely, Dr. Hahnemann left Leipsic in 1821 for Coethen. He stayed there until 1835 when he moved to Paris. While living in Coethen, he concentrated in attending almost exclusively to chronic disease cases. The outcome of this work was the development of a theory of chronic diseases, recorded in the book entitled " The Chronic Diseases, Their Peculiar Nature and Their Homeopathic Cure". It's first edition was published in 1828.

In the Author's Preface to the first edition of 1928, Dr. Hahnemann states: " If I did not know for what purpose I was put here on earth- to become better myself as far as possible and to make better everything around me, that is within my power to improve- I should have to consider myself as lacking very much in worldly prudence to make known for the common good, even before my death, an art which alone possess, and which it is within my power to make as profitable as possible by simply keeping it secret.

But in communicating to the world this great discovery, I am sorry that I must doubt whether my contemporaries will comprehend the logical sequence of these teachings of mine, and will follow them carefully and gain thereby the infinite benefits for suffering humanity which must inevitably spring from a faithful and accurate observance of the same; or whether, frightened away by the unheard of nature of many of these disclosures, they will not rather leave them untried and uninitiated and therefore useless.

And if they should not treat this discovery any better-well, then a more conscientious and intelligent posterity will alone have the advantage to be obtained by a faithful, punctual observance of the teachings here laid down, of being able to deliver mankind from the numberless torments which have rested upon the poor sick, owing to the numberless, tedious diseases, even as far back as history extends." *1

Dr. Hahnemann systematized his homeopathic system of healing in three major scientific publications: The Organon of Medicine (he considered the six edition to be "the most nearly perfect of all") *2, The Chronic Diseases, Their Peculiar Nature and Their Homeopathic Cure, and the Materia Medica Pura.

Chief among his remarkable new system of medicine was his the theory of chronic illness and crucial among its findings was the concept of miasms.

Yasgur's Homeopathic Dictionary defines miasms as " a noxious influence". *3

Miasms have been at the center of Dr. Hahnemann's work on chronic diseases. He notices that individuals that have been treated and cured of chronic conditions, later on this conditions would re-appear; sometime within months, others within years. He realized that something else played a part in these re-occurrences and later on he was able to discover that they were caused by specific inherited or acquired factors that he called Miasms and that the remedies that temporarily eliminated the condition where homeopathic to the symptoms but not to these miasms.

Dr. Hahnemann pointed out an important difference between acute miasmatic diseases and chronic miasmatic ones. In acute diseases the human constitution has the ability to cure them in a short time by his own organism; unless it is of such an intensity or has complications that may ended up killing him. Chronic miasmatic diseases shared the same causation/contagion and the formation of the internal disease before any external manifestations. However, the crucial difference of chronic miasmatic diseases with acute one is that in the chronic miasmata the internal disease remains in the organism during the entire life and increases every year, unless it is eliminated by the appropriate homeopathic treatment.

He believed that we have been endowed with a vital force that has the property and power to keep us healthy throughout the life process. However, this vital force is not able by itself to achieve cure without the assistance of remedies, even though he acknowledges that when thus assisted, the vital force is the conqueror of illnesses, not the remedies. This vital force is "only sufficient to maintain the unimpeded progress of life." *4

The above, he said, was particularly true when dealing with chronic diseases. He believed that only homeopathic medicine can give the life force the power it needs to overcome them. He theorized that by " itself the vital principle, being only an organic vital force intended to preserve an undisturbed health, opposes only a weak resistance to the invading morbific enemy; as the disease grows and increases, it opposes a greater resistance, but at best it is only an equal resistance; with weakly patients it is not even equal, but weaker."*5

Dr. Hahnemann stated that: "…the fundamental essence of this spiritual vital principle, imparted to us men by the infinitely merciful Creator, is incredibly great, if we physicians understand how to maintain its integrity in days of health, by directing men to a healthy mode of living, and how to invoke and augment it in diseases by purely homeopathic treatment." *6

At the core of homeopathy is the process of dynamization by which the medicinal properties of a substance which are latent in its crude form comes forth and become able to function " in an almost spiritual manner on our life". *7

This dynamization process brings forth the true essence of the medicinal substance which will expose its most " subtle part" of its medicinal powers. *8

An important parallel must be point out between how the process of dynamization breaks thru the layers of crude substance in order to find its healing powers and Dr. Bach's flower essences designed to break through the layers within a being in order to release the healing power within " the soul".

Dr. Hahnemann acknowledged that homeopaths were able to remove chronic diseases with remedies available at that time and that these cures far excelled those of allopaths. However, sometimes the cured diseased will come back and he notice that : " Even some gross errors of diet, taking cold, the appearance of weather especially rough, wet and cold or stormy, or even the approach of autumn, if ever so mild, but, more yet, winter and a wintry spring, and then some violent exertion of the body or mind, but particularly some shock to the health caused by some severe external injury, or a very sad event that bowed down the soul, repeated fright, great grief, sorrow and continuous vexation, often caused in a weakened body the re-appearance of one or more of the ailments which seemed to have been already overcome; and this new condition was often aggravated by some quite new concomitants, which if not more threatening than the former one which has been removed homeopathically were often just as troublesome and now more obstinate." *9

He noticed that this was often the case when you were dealing with chronic illnesses that have as their foundation the psoric miasm more fully developed or manifested. This happened because the homeopathic remedies given to cured the original condition was homeopathic to the symptoms of the chronic condition but not to the miasmatic root of the disease.

First he thought that it was because they did not have a sufficient number of remedies, but as these numbers increased there was still no cure for the psoric (non- venereal) based chronic illnesses. The vital force assisted by homeopathic remedies was not able to overcome these conditions. Trying to understand what prevented its cure led him to develop his theory on chronic diseases. He dedicated two years (1816 and 1817) of his life to solve this puzzle. He waited until 1827 to disclosed this discovery to two of his most trusted students in order for it not to be lost.

It was, as he stated, " a continually repeated fact that the non-venereal chronic diseases, after being time and again removed homeopathically by the remedies fully proven up to the present time, always returned in a more or less varied form and with new symptoms, or reappeared annually with an increases of complaints." Consequently the physician not only had to treat the present disease, but also the "separate fragment of a more deep-seated original disease". *10

The physician " must first find out as far as possible the whole extent of all the accidents and symptoms belonging to the unknown primitive malady before he come to discover one or more medicines which may homeopathically cover the whole of the original disease by means of its peculiar symptoms. The original malady sought for must be also of a miasmatic, chronic nature...that after it has once advanced to a certain degree it can never be removed by the strength of any robust constitution, it can never be overcome by the most wholesome diet and order of life, nor will it die out of itself." *11

He believed that throughout the world there were three chronic miasms: Shyphilis, also called the venereal changre disease; Sycosis, or the fig-wart disease and Psora, which lies at the foundation of itch.

PSORA

To Psora he attributed not only the many cutaneous eruptions but other conditions and thousands diseases such as:
- Common wart on the finger
- Sarcomatous tumor
- Finger-nails malformations
- Swelling of the bones
- Curvature of the spine
- Many deformities of the bones
- Frequent epistaxis
- The accumulation of blood in the veins of the rectum and the anus
- Discharges of blood from the rectum and anus
- Blind or flowing piles
- Hemoptysis
- Hematemesis
- Hematuria
- Deficient as well as too frequent menstrual discharges
- Night sweats of several years duration
- Parchment-like dryness of the skin
- Diarrhea of many years' standing
- Permanent constipation and difficult evacuation of the bowels
- Long-continued erratic pains.

- Convulsions occurring repeatedly for a number of years
- Chronic ulcers and inflammation
- Sarcomatous enlargements and tumors
- Emaciation
- Excessive sensitiveness as well as deficiencies in the senses of seeing, hearing, smelling, tasting and feeling
- Excessive as well as extinguished sexual desire
- Diseases of the mind and of the soul, from imbecility up to ecstacy, from melancholy up to raging insanity
- Swoons and vertigo
- Diseases of the heart Abdominal complaints
- All that is comprehended under hysteria and hypochondria
- And thousands of others illnesses
- Gout
- Consumption
- Tubercular phthisis
- Continual or spasmodic asthma
- Blindness
- Deafness
- Paralysis
- Osteoporosis
- Ulcers
- Cancer
- Spasms
- Hemorrhages
- Suffocating catarrh
- Pleurisy
- Degeneration of the brain
- Cataract
- Piles
- Diabetes
- Erysipelas
- Apoplexy
- Paralysis
- Melancholy
- Insanity, etc.

According to Dr. Proceso Sanchez Ortega, " psora is an imbalance due to deficiency, to insufficiency, inhibition, to an alteration in rhythm in the sense of less, all the organs and their cells producing insufficiency." *12

Dr. Hahnemann believed, based on his personal observations that "the ailments and infirmities of body and soul which, in their manifest complaints, differ so radically and which, with different patients, appear so very unlike (if they do not belong to the two veneral diseases, syphilis and sycosis), are but partial manifestations of the ancient miasma of leprosy and itch; e.g., merely descendants of one and the same vast original malady, the almost innumerable symptoms of which form but one whole and are to be regarded and to be medicinally treated as the parts of one and the same disease in the same way as in a great epidemic of typhus fever." *13

He believed that Pora was the most ancient of all chronic miasms. In his attempt to identify its point of origin in history he finds that it preceded all recorded history. Throughout history Psora had different names: leprosy, itch, erysipelas, etc. He points out that when Psora appeared in the form of leprosy, the condition was very much controlled by the mere fact that lepers were isolated and thus infection was limited. Furthermore, leprosy was very difficult for those suffering from it because of the external manifestations on the skin but they shared a fair level of general health. However, the very milder form of Psora during the fourteenth and fifteenth centuries when it appeared as itch, the few pustules after an infection could be easily covered but due to the fluid emitted after scratching infections became more widely spread.

With the different treatments repressing the itch, Psora grows more within, without the external skin eruption, but causing a legion of other diseases that to this date allopathic practitioners created an endless list of individual diseases, chronic and acute that have this hidden Psoric miasm at their root which are treated by innumerable suppressive methods that further drives Psora within and setting the stage to further diseases with the same miasmatic root.

This is how Psora became the most ancient, infectious and most general of all chronic miams to the extend that it is believed that there is only one true miasm without which the others could not exist and Psora is this miasm. It became, as Hahnemann said, " the most universal mother of chronic diseases." *14. Psora became to be recognized as the miasm that provided the framework for all other miasms.

With respect to the origin of the three chronic miasms: psoric, sycotic and syphilitic, Hahnemann states: " As in the acute, miasmatic eruptional diseases, three different important moments are to be attentively considered than the hitherto been done: First, the time of infection; secondly, the period of time during which the whole organism is being penetrated by the disease infused, until it has developed within; and thirdly, the breaking out of the external ailment, whereby nature externally demonstrates the completion of the internal development of the miasmatic malady throughout the whole organism". *15

(Note:The issue of how miasms are acquired has been debated since Dr. Hahnemann first offered his theory of chronic diseases to the world. Opinions ranged from being acquired via an infection, inherited, to a vibrational imbalance,etc. Dr. Tomas Pablo Paschero believed that " a miasm is not an infection or an intoxication but a vibratory alteration of man's vital energy determining the biological behavior and genetic constitution of the individual." *16).

With reference to the mode of contagion among chronic miasms, Hanemann states: "the itch disease (Psora) is, however the most contagious of all chronic miasmata, far more infectious than the other two chronic miasmata, the venereal chancre disease (syphilis) and the fig-wart disease (sycosis). To effect the infection with the latter it is required a certain amount of friction in the most tender parts of the body, which are the most rich in nerves and covered with the thinnest cuticle, as in the genital organs, unless the miasma should touch a wounded spot. But the miasma of the itch needs only to touch the general skin especially with tender children. The disposition of being affected with the miasma of itch is found with almost everyone and under almost all circumstance, which is not the case with the other two miasmata." *17

SYMPTOMS OF LATENT PSORA:
- Frequent discharge of ascarides and other worms; unsufferable itching caused by the latter in the rectum
- The abdomen often distended

- Now insatiable hunger, then again want of appetite
- Paleness of the face and relaxation of the muscles
- Frequent inflammation of the eyes
- Swelling of the cervical glands
- Perspiration on the head, in the evening after going to sleep
- Epistaxis with girls and youths
- Usually cold hands or perspiration on the palms
- The arms or hands, the legs or feet, are benumbed by a slight cause
- Frequent cramps in the calves, the muscles of the arms and hands
- Painless subsultus of various portions of the muscles here and there on the body
- Frequent or tedious dry or fluent coryza or catarrh, or impossibility of catching a cold or even from the most severe exposure
- Long continued obstruction of one or both nostrils
- Ulcerated nostrils
- Disagreeable sensation of dryness in the nose
- Frequent inflammation of the throat, frequent hoarseness
- Short tussiculation in the morning
- Frequent attacks of dyspnoea
- Predisposition to catching cold either in the whole body or in parts, such as chest, head, etc.
- Predispositions to strains, even from carrying or lifting a slight weight
- Frequent one-sided headache or toothache
- Frequent flushes of heat and redness of the face
- Frequent falling of hair of the head, dryness of the same, many scales upon the scalps
- Irregularities of the menses
- Twitching of the limbs on going to sleep
- Weariness early on awaking; un-refreshing sleep
- Perspiration in the morning in bed
- Perspiration breaks out too easily during the daytime
- White or very pale tongue
- Much phlegm in the throat
- Sour taste in the mouth

- Nausea in the morning
- Sensation of emptiness in the stomach
- Repugnance to cooked, warm food
- Repugnance to milk
- Cutting pains in the abdomen
- Hard stools, usually covered with mucus
- Itching in the anus
- Dark urine
- Swollen, enlarged veins on the legs
- Disposition to crack, strain or wrench one joint or another
- Cracking of one or more joints on moving
- Uneasy, frightful, or al least too vivid, dreams
- Unhealthy skin
- Unbearably itching vesicle, sometimes filled with pus, causing burning sensation after rubbing
- Vertigo; reeling while walking
- Vertigo, when closing the eyes
- Vertigo, on turning around briskly
- Vertigo with frequent eructations
- Vertigo, when looking up or down
- Vertigo, resembling a swoon
- Vertigo, passing over into unconsciousness
- Dizziness
- Thoughts not under her/his control
- Headache, one side with periodicity
- Cold pressure on top of the head
- Throbbing headaches
- Roaring noise in the brain, singing, buzzing, humming, thundering, etc.
- Scalp full of dandruff, with or without itching
- Hair, frequently falling out
- Painful lumps under the skin
- Frequent redness and heat of the face
- Yellow color of the face
- Eyes, daylight sensitivity
- Eyes, edges full of dry mucus

- Eyes, inflammation
- Eyes, yellow of white of the eyes
- Eyes, dropsy
- Eyes, cataracts
- Eyes, false vision
- Eyes, night blindness
- Sensitive hearing
- Pulsation in the ear
- Deafness of various degrees
- Swelling of the parotid glands
- Polypi of the nose
- Sense of smell weak or lost
- Fetid smell in the nose
- Glandular swelling
- Gum bleeding at a slight touch
- Gum recession
- Gnashing of the teeth during sleep
- Looseness of the teeth
- Tongue, white coated
- Tongue full of deep furrows as if torn above
- Dry tongue
- Fetid smell from the mouth
- Frequent inflammation of the throat
- Bitter taste in the mouth
- Putrid and fetid taste in the mouth
- Eructations, with taste of the food several hours after eating
- Eructations, incomplete, sour, rancid, etc.
- Hearburn
- Nausea early in the morning
- Nausea always after eating fatty things or milk
- Vomiting of blood
- Ravenous hunger
- Want of appetite
- Stomach, griping, pain in the pit of the stomach, spasm, pressure
- After eating, anxiety and cold perspiration with anxiety
- Distention of the abdomen after eating

- After meals, very tired, headache, palpitation of the heart
- Liver, inflammation and pain
- Constipation
- Stools, very pale, whitish, green, gray, clay- colored
- Frequent repeated diarrhea
- Painful retention of the urine
- Cannot hold the urine
- Frequent micturition at night
- Urine, dark yellow, turbid like whey, brown, blackish, with blood particles
- Lack of sexual desire or uncontrollable insatiable lasciviousness
- Disorders of the menstrual function
- Sterility, impotence without organic cause
- Premature births
- Freckles
- Liver spots
- Sleep disorders
- Vivid dreams
- Somnambulism
- Disturbances of the mind and spirit of all kinds
- Mania of self destruction
- Melancholy
- Anxiety
- Excessive sensitiveness
- Irritability from weakness
- Etc.*18

The above symptoms were some of the symptoms that Dr. Hahnemann identified as manifestation of latent Psora, which if repeated or became constant will indicate that the internal Psora is coming forth from its latent state. These symptoms are not the expression of any particular disease, they indicate the presence of Psora and if it is not properly treated it will later on break out in disastrous ways.

SYCOSIS

Sycosis was recognized by Dr. Hahnemann for its production of neoformations, with dentated growths resembling figs. This is a pathological condition of excess. According to him, this was a miasmata that produced the fewest chronic diseases. This figwart-disease was usually treated with mercury because it was considered similar to the venereal chancre-disease. The excrescenses on the genital were treated allopathically very aggressively by cauterizing, burning, cutting or by ligatures; thus driving the condition further inside. This miasm is expressed in various forms:

- A tendency for making a secret of everything
- Anxiety about its secrecy
- Suspicious of everybody and everything
- Tendency for brooding over things
- The sycotic mind is grossly debased
- It makes the memory weaker and weaker, particularly with respect to names and dates.
- The sycotic mind is suspicious, mischievous, mean, selfish and forgetful
- Tendency for condylomatous growths of various sizes and colours
- All tumors and tumorous growths
- All unusual fleshy growths, piles
- Extremely irritable temper
- Tendency for frequent urination
- Poverty of language and thought
- Pain is changing, erratic, stabbing, unbearable
- Must always be on the move, changing position, finding another place
- Constantly in an uproar, applying himself to numerous projects
- He is precipitate
- Always wanting something and pursuing it
- Audacious, the classic winner
- Specific indications such as:
  - Inflammation of the testes
  - Arthritis
  - Rheumatism
  - Cold and catarrh in any part of the body (such as nose, throat, lung, stomach, etc.)
  - Anemia

- Emaciation of any part of the body
- All urinary troubles
- All uterine and ovarian troubles
- Teething troubles
- Sweating of the head, etc.

Sycosis is an anomalous constitutional state resulting from the arbitrary and unnatural suppression of acute illness characterized by fluxes and abundant secretions. Its constitutional pathology is demonstrated by a tendency to produce hyperplasias and hypertrophies. It constitutes a predisposition to excess and abnormal growths.

The mind is perverted and is thus projected into the body. The sychotic will typically wrap himself in a thick layer of fat; his perversion endows him with this exaggerated reserves and even prevents him from eliminating that which harms him.

This pathology will manifest the same tendency to accumulations in his bone structure such as arthritic nodes.

Always "in an uproar, will roam around various roads until dying in his physical and mental restlessness, in his excess, and his rapid wasting away, despite his great attachment to life." *19

SYPHILIS

Syphillis, the venereal chancre-disease was at the time of Hahnemann more widely spread than the figwart-disease. It is considered the worst of the exterminators of the human vital force. The original transgression causing psora becomes more all encompassing with the sycotic exaggeration, and with syphilis degenerated to extermination.

The specific manifestations of this miasm are:
- Violent in his reaction to society and others
- Full of rancor, hatred, the desire to kill or to commit suicide, fury, rage
- Cruelty, contempt for others, jealousy
- Night-time intensifies all imbalances

- Malignant abscesses and boils
- Fetid sweat
- Thick flabby tongue with a white coating and imprints teeth around the margin
- Severe pains in the bones, worse at night, in the heat of the bed
- Skin troubles are non-itching
- Intolerance to heat and cold
- Abnormal conditions of internal organs
- Headaches are worst at night
- Etc.

When syphilis, just acquired and manifested in the shape of an ulcer in the glands, is healed up by the accepted methods of treatment (injections, ointments, etc), it travels down into the interior of the body, resulting in a miasmatic infection of the very personality of the victim. Then it can come back in the shape of malignant buboes and later on in the shape of malignant abscesses and boils, until at last, it eats up the still finer tissues like the mucous membranes and bones.

Syphilis is very deep and insidious in its action, because it is not only the physical tissues that it attacks and destroys, but it also attacks the mind, and its characteristic way of expression of this attack is imbecility. This imbecility or idiocy is a slow, gradual process. With Psora the mind is over-active, with Sycosis is bad and with Syphilis is slow.

It must be pointed out that there are causes of chronic diseases that are making contemporary diseases more difficult to cure; causes that have aggravated the original miasmatic tendencies. Among them we find:

- Allopathic treatments and other suppressive methods of treatments
- Vaccinations and injections
- Gradual fineness and subtlety of the miasm as also knottiness of their bonds due to progressive heredity and uniting of directly acquired miasms with these hereditary forms
- Electromagnetic pollution
- All environmental pollution

- Geopathic stress
- Genetic modification of foods
- Etc.

These factors give us an idea of why the complexity of contemporary diseases and why we must rely on other methods of healing to correct these severely complex disease patterns. Of course there are other factors in addition to the ones stated above that continues to aggravate the extent of these diseases, making it indispensable the utilization of healing methods with high vibrational values with the ability to heal. Scientific literature and clinical experience demonstrate that Dr. Bach's flower essences are capable of performing this level of healing without negative side effects, healing crisis or aggravations.

Dr. Hahnemann found Psora to be the oldest most pervasive of all miasms. Dr. Bach went beyond these disease facilitators and identified the ultimate cause of disease: a conflict between the soul and the mind and build around these finding a new system of healing.

Dr. Bach believed that his new system of healing advanced Dr. Hahnemann's work in homeopathy. This may appeared to be a fundamental contradiction since his new system of healing did not use homeopathic remedies. However, this is not so.

First, Dr. Bach, as Dr. Hahnemann, seeing the great limitations of allopathic medicine, was looking for a new healing system. Dr. Bach found one that was new, simple and accessible to all in their own homes.

Secondly, Dr. Bach, as Dr. Hahnemann, discovered a system of healing that was both free of harmful side effects and healing at the same time.

Thirdly, Dr. Bach's, as Dr. Hahnemann's, was a system of healing based on the vibrational properties of the chosen remedies. His method, following the basic scientific principles of homeopathy, advanced its cause by its simplicity, effectiveness and accessibility to the general population.

Even though, Dr. Bach went beyond miasm in the identification of the origin of diseases, miasmatic tendencies is a scientific reality and his method is very relevant in the modification of these tendencies that are at the root of some many acute and chronic conditions. His system of healing offers a simple, speedy and effective way to treat them without any adverse effect, such as healing crisis.

*1   Hahnemann, Dr., Samuel, *The Chronic Diseases- Their Peculiar Nature and Their Homeopathic Cure*, (B. Jain Publishers, Ltd., India, 2001), Author's Preface to the first edition- 1828

*2   Hahnemann, Dr., Samuel, *Organon of Medicine,* (B. Jain Publishers, Ltd, India, 1997), Translator's Preface, p.3.

*3   Yasgur, Jay, *Yasgur Homeopathic Dictionary,*(Van Hoy Publishers, Pa, USA, 2004), p.153

*4   Hahnemann, Dr., Samuel, *The Chronic Diseases- Theoretical Part,* (B. Jain Publishers, Ltd, India, 2004), p.13

*5   Hahnemann, Dr., Samuel, *The Chronic Diseases- Their Peculiar Nature and Their Homeopathic Cure,*(B. Jain Publishers, Ltd, India, 2001), p.xviii

*6   Hahnemann, Dr., Samuel, *The Chronic Diseases-Their Peculiar Nature and Their Homeopathic Cure,* (B. Jain Publishers, Ltd., India, 2001), p.xix

*7   Hahnemann, Dr., Samuel, *The Chronic Diseases- Their Peculiar Nature and Their Homeopathic Cure,* (B. Jain Publishers, Ltd., India, 2001), p.xix

*8   Hahnemann, Dr., Samuel, *The Chronic Diseases- Their Peculiar Nature and Their Homeopathic Cure,* (B. Jain Publishers, Ltd., India, 2001), p. xix

*9   Hahnemann, Dr., Samuel, *The Chronic Diseases- Their Peculiar Nature and Their Homeopathic Cure,* (B. Jain Publishers, Ltd., India, 2001), p.3

*10   Hahnemann, Dr., Samuel, *The Chronic Diseases- Their Peculiar Nature and Their Homeopathic Cure,* (B. Jain Publishers, Ltd., India, 2001), p.5

*11   Hahnemann, Dr., Samuel, *The Chronic Diseases- Their Peculiar Nature and Their Homeopathic Cure,* (B. Jain Publishers, Ltd., India, 2001), p.6

*12   Ortega-Sanchez, Dr., Proceso, *Notes on the Miasms or Hahnemann's Chronic Diseases*, (Published by the National Homeopathic Pharmacy, New Dehli, India, 1980), p.63

*13   Hahnemann, Dr., Samuel, *The Chronic Diseases- Their Peculiar Nature and Their Homeopathic Cure,* (B. Jain Publishers, Ltd., India, 2001, p.8

*14   Hahnemann, Dr., Samuel, *The Chronic Diseases- Their Peculiar Nature and Their Homeopathic Cure*, (B. Jain Publishers, Ltd., India, 2001), p.13

*15   Hahnemann, Dr., Samuel, *The Chronic Diseases- Their Peculiar Nature and Their Homeopathic Cure*, (B. Jain Publishers, Ltd., India, 2001), p.33

*16   Mathur, Dr., K.N., *Principles of Prescribing- Collected from Clinical Experiences of Pioneers of Homeopathy*, (B. Jain Publishers, Ltd., India, 2006), p.175

*17   Hahnemann, Dr., Samuel, *The Chronic Diseases- Their Peculiar Nature and Their Homeopathic Cure*, (B. Jain Publishers, Ltd., India, 2001), p.37

*18   Hahnemann, Dr., Samuel, *The Chronic Diseases- Their Peculiar Nature and Their Homeopathic Cure*, (B. Jain Publishers, Ltd., India, 2001), pp. 45-79

*19   Ortega-Sanchez, Dr., Proceso, *Notes on the Miasms or Hahnemann's Chronic Diseases*, (Published by the National Homeopathic Pharmacy, New Dehli, India, 1980), p.71

PROTOCOLS

" The mind must be healed first and the body will follow."
Dr. Edward Bach

PROTOCOLS

The following protocols were identified via radiesthesia, thus unique to each individual and should not be interpreted or prescribed to others with similar chronic/miasmatic conditions or other conditions listed under Miscellaneous Protocols.

These protocols are included to illustrate the range of conditions that can be treated exclusively with Bach's Flower Essences. Just as Dr. Bach indicated, they can cure all illnesses/imbalances.

Under Miscellaneous Protocols more examples are included under negative cell memories, constitutional strength, mental/emotional imbalances, and detoxification. These are given to assist the practitioner to look beyond the obvious conditionand get to the root of the problem. Very often these areas are behind the expressed or physically manifested symptoms.

All conditions whether acute or chronic are rooted somewhere hidden from the physical condition. Furthermore you can have clients with the same physical manifestation, in the same part of the body, with the same characteristics and modalities and each will required a different formula. Access to the quantum field via radiesthesia will grant the practitioner the venue to get to the root of the problem and the sequence of treatment to re-established harmony throughout the client's entire being.

This author prefers to address conditions as imbalances, since illnesses are imbalances. Correct the imbalance and the client will be restored to health/ harmony.

The author included only cases that were resolved with flower essences only.

As a general guideline, the practitioner needs to:

a) Identify the pattern of imbalance

b) Assess/ quantify the degree of severity of condition in order to later measure the degree of progress.

c) Identify the first flower essence protocol

d) Determine the dosage

e) After initial protocol is completed, the practitioner needs to test the degree of condition resolution in order to determine the next step.

Bach's Flower Essences are excellent facilitators of healing and the client's cooperation is crucial to achieve the self healing he/she needs.

AUTHOR'S CLINICAL CASES

" The action of these remedies is to raise our vibrations and open up the channels for the reception of our spiritual self, to flood our natures with the particular virtue we need and wash out from us the fault which is causing harm." Dr. Edward Bach

ANTI-MIASMATIC PROTOCOLS

" Disease lies in our own personality and it is within our own control." Dr. Edward Bach

ANTI-MIASMATIC PROTOCOLS

The following anti-miasmatic protocols were formulated to modify the individual miasmatic tendencies of the client. Other formulas may be subsequently needed in order to deal with the residual effects of these tendencies on the body, mind, emotion, cellular memory, etc. if they remain present after the original anti-miasmatic protocol was completed.

Unless otherwise indicated, all dose drops are from compounded formulas.

PSORIC MIASM:

1.   CLIENT: Middle Age Female

       FLOWER ESSENCES: Clematis
                               Heather
                               Rock Rose
                               Scleranthus
                               Rescue Remedy

       FORMULA: 1 oz. of water in a dropper bottle
                               4 drops of each of the selected
                               flower essences
                               Potentized 11 times
       RX: 5 drops **, 2 times per day for 11

days.

2.   CLIENT: Elderly Female

    FLOWER ESSENCES: Cherry Plum
Gentian
Sweet Chestnut
Willow
Rescue Remedy

    FORMULA: 1 oz. of water in a dropper bottle
5 drops of each of the selected
flower essences

    RX: 4 drops, 3 times per day for 7
days

3.   CLIENT: Middle Age Female

    FLOWER ESSENCES: Agrimony
Impatiens
Larch
Pine
Vervain
Rescue Remedy

    FORMULA: 1 oz. of water in a dropper bottle
5 drops of each of the selected
flower essences

    RX: 5 drops, three times per day for
10 days

4.   CLIENT: Young Male

    FLOWER ESSENCES: Vine

		Red Chestnut Rock Rose Rescue Remedy
	FORMULA:	1 oz. of water in a dropper bottle 5 drops of each of the selected flower essences Potentized 5 times
	RX:	3 drops, 2 times per day for 9 days
5.	CLIENT:	Middle-Age Female
	FLOWER ESSENCES:	Cherry Plum Red Chestnut Rescue Remedy
	FORMULA:	1 oz. of water in a dropper bottle 3 drops of each of the selected flower essences
	RX:	5 drops, 3 times per day for 8 days.
6.	CLIENT:	Middle-Age Female
	FLOWER ESSENCES:	Impatiens Vervain Rock Rose Rescue Remedy
	FORMULA:	1 oz. of water in a dropper bottle 5 drops of each of the selected flower essences
	RX:	5 drops, 2 times per day for 7

days.

7.   CLIENT: Young Girl

FLOWER ESSENCES:
Larch
Red Chestnut
Vine
Rescue Remedy

FORMULA:
1 oz of water in a dropper bottle
5 drops of each of the selected
flower essences

RX:
3 drops, 2 times per day for 5
days

8.   CLIENT: Middle-Age Female

FLOWER ESSENCES:
Red Chestnut
Rock Rose
Rock Water
Sweet Chestnut
Vine
Rescue Remedy

FORMULA:
1 oz. of water in a dropper bottle
4 drops of each of the selected
flower essences

RX:
4 drops, 3 times per day for 6
days

9.   CLIENT: Middle-Age Female

FLOWER ESSENCES:
Agrimony
Centaury

	Olive Rock Water Star of Bethlehem Vine Rescue Remedy
FORMULA:	1 oz. of water in a dropper bottle 4 drops of each of the selected flower essences except for 8 drops of Olive.
RX:	4 drops, 3 times per day for 35 days.
10. CLIENT:	Female Cat
FLOWER ESSENCES:	Clematis Olive Pine Rescue Remedy
FORMULA:	1 oz of water in a dropper bottle 5 drops of each of the selected flower essences
RX:	4 drops, 2 times per day for 3 days
11. CLIENT:	Female Dog
FLOWER ESSENCES:	Vine Walnut Water Violet Rescue Remedy
FORMULA:	1 oz. of water in a dropper bottle

		3 drops of each of the selected flower essences
	RX:	4 drops, 2 times per day for 4 days

12.	CLIENT:	Female Cat
	FLOWER ESSENCES:	Sweet Chestnut White Chestnut Rescue Remedy
	FORMULA:	1 oz. of water in a dropper bottle 3 drops of each of the selected flower essences
	RX:	3 drops, 2 times per day for 3 days

SYCOTIC MIASM:

1.	CLIENT:	Young Male
	FLOWER ESSENCES:	Agrimony Honeysuckle Vervain Water Violet Rescue Remedy
	FORMULA:	1 oz. of water in a dropper bottle 3 drops of each of the selected flower essences
	RX:	4 drops, 2 times per day for 10 days
2.	CLIENT:	Young Female

<table>
<tr><td></td><td>FLOWER ESSENCES:</td><td>Scleranthus
Rock Rose
Rock Water
Rescue Remedy</td></tr>
<tr><td></td><td>FORMULA:</td><td>1 oz. of water in a dropper bottle
5 drops of each of the selected
flower essences</td></tr>
<tr><td></td><td>RX:</td><td>3 drops, 4 times per day for 9
days</td></tr>
<tr><td>3.</td><td>CLIENT:</td><td>Middle-Age Female</td></tr>
<tr><td></td><td>FLOWER ESSENCES:</td><td>Rock Water
Sweet Chestnut
Rescue Remedy</td></tr>
<tr><td></td><td>FORMULA:</td><td>1 oz. of water in a dropper bottle
5 drops of each of the selected
flower essences</td></tr>
<tr><td></td><td>RX:</td><td>3 drops, 2 times per day for 6
days</td></tr>
<tr><td>4.</td><td>CLIENT:</td><td>Elderly Male</td></tr>
<tr><td></td><td>FLOWER ESSENCES:</td><td>Gorse
Vine
Wild Oat
Rescue Remedy</td></tr>
<tr><td></td><td>FORMULA:</td><td>1 oz. of water in a dropper bottle</td></tr>
</table>

		5 drops of each of the selected flower essences
	RX:	4 drops, 2 times per day for 7 days

5.	CLIENT:	Middle-Age Female
	FLOWER ESSENCES:	Agrimony Beech Cerato Willow Rescue Remedy
	FORMULA:	1 oz. of water in a dropper bottle 4 drops of each of the selected flower essences
	RX:	3 drops, 2 times per day for 12 days

6.	CLIENT:	Young Male
	FLOWER ESSENCES:	Larch Vervain Vine Rescue Remedy
	FORMULA:	1 oz. of water in a dropper bottle 5 drops of each of the selected flower essences
	RX:	5 drops, 3 times per day for 7 days

7.	CLIENT:	Young Female

FLOWER ESSENCES:	White Chestnut Rescue Remedy
FORMULA:	1 oz. of water in a dropper bottle 6 drops of each of the selected flower essences
RX:	4 drops, 3 times per day for 14 days

8.

CLIENT:	Middle-Age Female
FLOWER ESSENCES:	Gorse Honeysuckle Hornbeam Rescue Remedy
FORMULA:	1 oz. of water in a dropper bottle 5 drops of each of the selected flower essences
RX:	4 drops, 2 times per day for 8 days

9.

CLIENT:	Middle-Age Male
FLOWER ESSENCES:	Aspen Walnut Rescue Remedy
FORMULA:	1 oz. of water in a dropper bottle 5 drops of each of the selected flower essences
RX:	4 drops, 2 times per day for 5

days

10. CLIENT: Young Female

FLOWER ESSENCES: Mimulus
Rescue Remedy

FORMULA: None

RX: 3 drops of each of the selected
flower essences from
the stock bottle, 2 times per day
for 4 days

11. CLIENT: Young Female Cat

FLOWER ESSENCES: Impatiens
Rescue Remedy

FORMULA: 1 oz. of water in a dropper bottle
3 drops of each of the selected
flower essences

RX: 3 drops, 2 times per day for 3
days

12. CLIENT: Adult Male Dog

FLOWER ESSENCES: Mimulus
Rescue Remedy

FORMULA: 1 oz. of water in a dropper bottle
2 drops of each of the selected
flower essences

RX: 2 drops, 2 times per day for 5

days

SYPHILITIC MIASM

1.   CLIENT: Young Female

       FLOWER ESSENCES: Clematis
Crab Apple
Mustard
Sweet Chestnut
Vine
Water Violet
Rescue Remedy

       FORMULA: 1oz. of water in a dropper bottle
5 drops of each of the selected
flower essences

       RX: 4 drops, 2 times per day for 8
days

2.   CLIENT: Young Male

       FLOWER ESSENCES: Agrimony
Crab Apple
Mimulus
Willow
Rescue Remedy

       FORMULA: 1 oz. of water in a dropper bottle

                                  5 drops of each of the selected
flower essences

       RX: 5 drops, 2 times per day for 4

		days
3.	CLIENT:	Young Female
	FLOWER ESSENCES:	Hornbeam Water Violet Rescue Remedy
	FORMULA:	None
	RX:	Hornbeam: 5 drops, 2 times per day for 5 days; followed by Water Violet: 5 drops, 2 times per day for 5 days; followed by Rescue Remedy, 5 drops, 2 times per day for 5 days.
4.	CLIENT:	Middle-Age Female
	FLOWER ESSENCES:	Elm Gentian Mustard Vine Walnut Rescue Remedy
	FORMULA:	1 oz. of water in a dropper bottle 5 drops of each of the selected flower essences Potentized 5 times
	RX:	3 drops, 2 times per day for 5 days
5.	CLIENT:	Middle-Age Male
	FLOWER ESSENCES:	Heather

		Hornbeam Rock Water Rescue Remedy
	FORMULA:	1 oz. of water in a dropper bottle 5 drops of each of the selected flower essences
	RX:	4 drops, 2 times per day for 9 days
6.	CLIENT:	Young Female
	FLOWER ESSENCES:	Centaury Gorse Rescue Remedy
	FORMULA:	1 oz. of water in a dropper bottle 5 drops of each of the selected flower essences Potentized 8 times
	RX:	4 drops, 2 times per day for 8 days
7.	CLIENT:	Middle-Age Female
	FLOWER ESSENCES:	Beech Rescue Remedy
	FORMULA:	1 oz, of water in a dropper bottle 5 drops of each of the selected flower essences
	RX:	3 drops of each, 3 times per day

for 10 days

8.   CLIENT: Middle-Age Female

FLOWER ESSENCES: Larch
Rescue Remedy

FORMULA: 1 oz. of water in a dropper bottle
4 drops of each of the selected
flower essences

RX: 3 drops, 3 times per day for 7
days

9.   CLIENT: Middle-Age Female

FLOWER ESSENCES: Centaury
Chestnut Bud
Elm
Rescue Remedy

FORMULA: 1 oz of water in a dropper bottle
3 drops of each of the selected
flower essences

RX: 5 drops, 2 times per day for 8
days

10.   CLIENT: Middle-Age Female

FLOWER ESSENCES: Cerato
Chestnut Bud
Aspen
Rescue Remedy

FORMULA: 1 oz. of water in a dropper bottle

		4 drops of Cerato and Chestnut Bud, 8 drops of Aspen and 5 drops of Rescue Remedy
	RX:	7 drops, 2 times per day for 2 weeks
11.	CLIENT:	Young Female Cat
	FLOWER ESSENCES:	Elm Rescue Remedy
	FORMULA:	1 oz. of water in a dropper bottle 3 drops of each of the selected flower essences
	RX:	3 drops, 2 times per day for 3 days
12.	CLIENT:	Elderly Female Cat
	FLOWER ESSENCES:	Gentian Gorse Impatiens Rock Water Vine Rescue Remedy
	FORMULA:	1 oz. of water in a dropper bottle 3 drops of each of the selected flower essences, potentized 7 times
	RX:	3 drops, 2 times per day for 9 days

MISCELLANEOUS PROTOCOLS

" In life there are two kind of pain: bodily pain and thought pain, and of the two thought pain is the more grievous." Dr. Edward Bach

MISCELLANEOUS IMBALANCES/CONDITIONS

CONDITION	F/E	FORMULA	RX
AGGRESSION	WILD OAT WILD ROSE WILLOW	1OZ. OF WATER 5 DROPS OF EACH FLOWER ESENCE	5 DROPS 3 TIMES PER DAY FOR 4 DAYS
ALLERGY	ASPEN CHICORY CLEMATIS CRAB APPLE	1 OZ. OF WATER 5 DROPS OF EACH FLOWER ESSENCES 13 SUCUSSIONS	5 DROPS 3 TIMES PER DAY FOR 4 DAYS
ALLERGY	WILLOW RESCUE REMEDY	1 OZ. OF WATER 4 DROPS OF EACH FLOWER ESSENCE	3 DROPS 2 TIMES PER DAY FOR 3 DAYS
ALLERGY	CRAB APPLE	1 OZ. OF WATER 4 DROPS OF CRAB APPLE	4 DROPS 3 TIMES PER DAY FOR 4 DAYS
ARTHRITIS	HOLLY	1 OZ. OF WATER	

HONEYSUCKLE4 DROPS OF EACH
LARCH FLOWER ESSENCE
66 SUCCUSSIONS
RX: ACUTE STAGE: 4 DROPS EVERY 5 MINUTES, 2 TIMES; THEN
EVERY 20 MINUTES 3 TIMES; THEN EVERY HOUR 2 TIMES

BEHAVIOR MODIFICATION	GENTIAN RESCUE REMEDY	1 OZ.OF WATER 5 DROPS OF EACH FLOWER ESSENCE	5 DROPS 2 TIMES PER DAY FOR 3 DAYS
BLOOD PRESSURE	BEECH HORNBEAM		5 DROPS OF EACH 1 TIME
CELL MEMORY	CHERRY PLUM CHICORY OLIVE ROCK WATER	1 DROP OF EACH ON A BAND-AID; PLACE ON 3RD EYE FOR 24 HRS. CHANGE BAND-AID EVERY DAY. REPEAT FOR 11 DAYS	
CELL MEMORY	WATER VIOLET WHITE CHESTNUT WILD OAT WILLOW	1 OZ. OF WATER 4 GTT OF EACH FLOWER ESSENCE	3 DROPS 3 TIMES PER DAY FOR 4 DAYS
CELL MEMORY	AGRIMONY	1 OZ. OF WATER 4 DROPS OF AGRIMONY	4 DROPS 2 TIMES PER DAY FOR 3 DAYS
CELL MEMORY	MUSTARD SCLERANTHUS STAR OF BETHLEHEM WILD OAT WALNUT	1 OZ. OF WATER 4 DROPS OF EACH 42 SUCCUSSIONS	7 DROPS 2 TIMES PER DAY FOR 5 DAYS

WHITE CHESTNUT
WATER VIOLET

CELL MEMORY	CRAB APPLE	1 OZ. OF WATER 8 DROPS OF CRAB APPLE	4 DROPS 2 TIMES PER DAY FOR 5 DAYS
CELL MEMORY	HORNBEAM CLEMATIS WILLOW	1 OZ. OF WATER 4 DROPS OF EACH FLOWER ESSENCE 4 SUCCUSSIONS	4 DROPS 2 TIMES PER DAY FOR 8 DAYS
CELL MEMORY (PRE-BIRTH)	LARCH MIMULUS WILLOW	1 OZ. OF WATER 4 DROPS OF EACH FLOWER ESSENCE 67 SUCCUSSIONS	4DROPS 2 TIMES PER DAY FOR 5 DAYS
CELL MEMORY	CLEMATIS WILD OAT	1 OZ.WATER 4 DROPS OF EACH FLOWER ESSENCE	4 DROPS 2 TIMES PER DAY FOR 4 DAYS
CELL MEMORY	AGRIMONY	1 OZ. OF WATER 4 DROPS OF EACH FLOWER ESSENCE	4 DROPS 2 TIMES PER DAY FOR 3 DAYS
CELL MEMORY	AGRIMONY	1 OZ. WATER 2 DROPS OF EACH FLOWER ESSENCE	3 DROPS 2 TIMES PER DAY FOR 5 DAYS
CIRCULATION	BEECH	1 OZ OF WATER	5 DROPS

	CERATO	5 DROPS OF EACH	3 TIMES PER
	CHESTNUT BUD	FLOWER ESSENCE	DAY FOR
	LARCH		4 WEEKS
	MIMULUS		
	MUSTARD		
	OLIVE		
	STAR OF BETHLEHEM		
CONSTIPATION	CRAB APPLE	1 OZ. OF WATER	4 DROPS
		4 DROPS OF EACH	1 TIME PER
		FLOWER ESSENCE	DAY FOR
		75 SUCCUSSIONS	3 MONTHS
CONSTIPATION	MUSTARD	1 OZ WATER	4 DROPS
(ACUTE)	CRAB APPLE	4 DROPS OF EACH	EVERY 5
	RESCUE	FLOWER ESSENCE	MINUTES
	REMEDY	75 SUCCUSSIONS	5 TIMES
CONSTITUTION	MUSTARD	1 OZ OF WATER	4 DROPS
(IMBALANCE)	OAK	4 DROPS OF EACH	2 TIMES PER
	SCLERANTHUS		DAY FOR
			14 DAYS
CONSTITUTION	RED CHESTNUT	FROM THE STOCK	3 DROPS
(IMBALANCE)	VINE	BOTTLE	3 TIMES PER
	WALNUT		DAY FOR
	WATER VIOLET		7 DAYS
CONSTITUTION	HORNBEAM	FROM THE STOCK	3 DROPS OF
(ENHANCEMENT)	SWEET CHESTNUT	BOTTLE	EACH
	ROCK WATER		1 TIME PER
	WATER VIOLET		DAY FOR
			10 DAYS
CONSTITUTION	MUSTARD	1 OZ. OF WATER	4 DROPS

(ENHANCEMENT)	OAK SCLERANTHUS	4 DROPS OF EACH FLOWER ESSENCE 75 SUCCUSSIONS	2 TIMES PER DAY FOR 14 DAYS
CONSTITUTION (STRENGTHENING)	SCLERANTHUS WATER VIOLET WILD OAT WILLOW	1 OZ. OF WATER 4 DROPS OF EACH FLOWER ESSENCE	ACUTE: 4 DROPS EVERY 5 MINUTES 6 TIMES THEN: 4 DROPS 3 TIMES PER DAY FOR 6 WEEKS
CONSTITUTION (STRENGTHENING)	IMPATIENS ROCK ROSE SCLERANTHUS START OF BETHLEHEM	1 OZ OF WATER 5 DROPS OF EACH FLOWER ESSENCE	5 DROPS 2 TIMES PER DAY FOR 9 DAYS
CONSTITUTION (STRENGTHENING)	RESCUE REMEDY CLEMATIS CRAB APPLE GORSE MIMULUS OLIVE	1 OZ OF WATER 4 DROPS OF EACH FLOWER ESSENCE	3 DROPS 2 TIMES PER DAY FOR 14 DAYS
CONSTITUTION (STREGTHENING)	CENTAURY CHESTNUT BUD RED CHESTNUT VERVAIN	1 OZ.OF WATER 4 DROPS OF EACH FLOWER ESSENCE	4 DROPS 2 TIMES PER DAY FOR 7 DAYS
DEAFNESS	WILLOW	1 OZ OF WATER 4 DROPS OF FLOWER ESSENCE	3 DROPS 2 TIMES PER DAY FOR 5 DAYS
DEAFNESS	GORSE	1 OZ OF WATER	4 DROPS

	STAR OF	4 DROPS OF EACH	2 TIMES PER
	BETHLEHEM	FLOWER ESSENCE	DAY FOR
	WILD ROSE	12 SUCCUSSIONS	5 DAYS
DEAFNESS	HEATHER	1 OZ OF WATER	4 DROPS
	SCLERANTHUS	4 DROPS OF EACH	2 TIMES PER
		FLOWER ESSENCE	DAY FOR 9 DAYS
BIRTHPLACE	SCLERANTHUS	1 OZ OF WATER	4 DROPS
DETACHMENT	WALNUT	4 DROPS OF EACH	3 TIMES PER
	WATER VIOLET	FLOWER ESSENCE	DAY FOR
	WILD OAT	17 SUCCUSSIONS	3 DAYS
D-TOX	CLEMATIS	1 OZ OF WATER	3 DROPS
	CRAB APPLE	4 DROPS OF EACH	3 TIMES PER
	SCLERANTHUS	FLOWER ESSENCE	DAY FOR
	VINE		7 DAYS
	RESCUE REMEDY		
D-TOX	CRAB APPLE	1 OZ.OF WATER	3 DROPS
		4 DROPS OF	3 TIMES PER
		FLOWER ESSENCE	DAY FOR 4 DAYS
D- TOX	AGRIMONY	FROM THE STOCK	3 DROPS
(CAFFEINE)	CRAB APPLE	BOTTLE	2 TIMES
	ROCK ROSE		1 HOUR
	WILD OAT		APART
	RESCUE REMEDY		
D-TOX	RESCUE REMEDY	1 OZ OF WATER	5 DROPS

(TOXIC	AGRIMONY CLEMATIS MUSTARD OLIVE ROCK WATER SCLERANTHUS	OF EACH FLOWER ESSENCE 12 SUCCUSSIONS	2TIMES PER DAY FOR 7 DAYS
DEPRESSION	STAR OF BETHLEHEM	1OZ. OF WATER 4 DROPS OF FLOWER ESSENCE 75 SUCCUSSIONS	3 DROPS 2 TIMES PER DAY FOR 6 DAYS
DEPRESSION	WILD ROSE WILLOW RESCUE REMEDY	1 OZ OF WATER 4 DROPS OF EACH FLOWER ESSENCE 75 SUCCUSSIONS	3 DROPS 3 TIMES PER DAY FOR 3 DAYS
DEPRESSION	CHESTNUT BUD GORSE HEATHER HOLLY	1 OZ OF WATER 4 DROPS OF EACH FLOWER ESSENCE	4 DROPS 3 TIMES PER DAY FOR 17 DAYS
DEPRESSION	CLEMATIS RESCUE REMEDY	1 OZ OF WATER 8 DROPS OF EACH FLOWER ESSENCE	4 DROPS AS NEEDED
DEPRESSION	AGRIMONY ASPEN CHESTNUT BUD OLIVE	1 OZ OF WATER 3 DROPS OF EACH FLOWER ESSENCE	3 DROPS 3 TIMES PER DAY FOR 7 DAYS
DEPRESSION	RESCUE REMEDY MUSTARD	¼ OZ OF WATER 5 DROPS OF EACH FLOWER ESSENCE	5 DROPS 5 TIMES PER DAY FOR 2 DAYS
DIGESTION	LARCH	1 OZ OF WATER	3 DROPS

(DISORDER)	WILLOW	4 DROPS OF EACH FLOWER ESSENCE	2 TIMES PER DAY FOR 6 DAYS
DIZZINESS	SCLERANTHUS	1 OZ. OF WATER 5 DROPS OF EACH FLOWER ESSENCE 32 SUCCUSSIONS	5 DROPS 2 TIMES PER DAY FOR 10 DAYS
DREAMS (RECURRENT)	CLEMATIS ELM	1 OZ OF WATER 4 DROPS OF EACH FLOWER ESSENCE	4 DROPS 3 TIMES PER DAY FOR 4 DAYS
DREAM (NIGHTMARES)	CRAB APPLE	FROM THE STOCK BOTTLE	3 DROPS AT BED-TIME FOR 13 WEEKS
ECZEMA	MIMULUS ROCK WATER	1 OZ OF WATER 3 DROPS 2 DROPS 78 SUCCUSSIONS	3 DROPS 2 TIMES PER 1 DAY PER WEEK FOR 4 WEEKS
ECZEMA	CLEMATIS CRAB APPLE	FROM THE STOCK BOTTLE	4 DROPS OF EACH F/E 3 TIMES PER DAY FOR 10 DAYS
ECZEMA	CRAB APPLE IMPATIENS	1 OZ OF WATER 4 DROPS OF EACH FLOWER ESSENCE	3 DROPS 3 TIMES PER DAY FOR 5 DAYS
EMOTIONAL	ASPEN	1 OZ OF WATER	5 DROPS

IMBALANCE	BEECH STAR OF BETHLEHEM RESCUE REMEDY	5 DROPS OF EACH	3 TIMES PER DAY FOR 4 DAYS
EMOTIONAL IMBALANCE	RESCUE REMEDY WATER VIOLET VINE	1 OZ OF WATER 3 DROPS OF EACH FLOWER ESSENCE	3 DROPS 4 TIMES PER DAY FOR 14 DAYS
EMOTIONAL IMBALANCE	IMPATIENS MIMULUS SWEET CHESTNUT WILLOW RESCUE REMEDY	1 OZ OF WATER 4 DROPS OF EACH FLOWER ESSENCE 26 SUCCUSSIONS	4 DROPS AS NEEDED
EQUILIBRIUM (MOTOR)	SCLERANTHUS WILLOW RESCUE REMEDY	1 OZ OF WATER 4 DROPS OF EACH FLOWER ESSENCE 75 SUCCUSSIONS	2 DROPS 2 TIMES PER DAY FOR 12 DAYS
EQUILIBRIUM (MOTOR)	SCLERANTHUS	1 OZ OF WATER 4 DROPS OF FLOWER ESSENCE	4 DROPS 3 TIMES PER DAY FOR 21 DAYS
EQUILIBRIUM (MOTOR)	CRAB APPLE GENTIAN PINE SCLERANTHUS	1 OZ OF WATER 4 DROPS OF EACH FLOWER ESSENCE	4 DROPS 4 TIMES PER DAY FOR 9 DAYS
EQUILIBRIUM (MOTOR)	RESCUE REMEDY CHESTNUT BUD MIMULUS SCLERANTHUS	1 OZ OF WATER 4 DROPS OF EACH FLOWER ESSENCE 15 SUCCUSSIONS	3 DROPS 2 TIMES PER DAY FOR 7 DAYS
EXHAUSTION	VINE	3 DROPS EVERY 15 MINUTES, 2 TIMES	

RESCUE REMEDY 4 DROPS EVERY 10 MINUTES, 2 TIMES

FEAR	WILLOW ROCK ROSE	1 OZ OF WATER 5 DROPS OF EACH FLOWER ESSENCE	3 DROPS AS NEEDED
FEAR	OLIVE STAR OF BETHLEHEM	1 OZ OF WATER 4 DROPS OF EACH FLOWER ESSENCE	4 DROPS 2 TIMES PER DAY FOR 21 DAYS
FEAR	RED CHESTNUT	5 DROPS	2 TIMES PER DAY FOR 7 DAYS
FISTULA (GUM)	CRAB APPLE	FROM THE STOCK BOTTLE	1 DROP 1 TIME PER DAY FOR 3 DAYS
FLU	 RESCUE REMEDY CHICORY CHERRY PLUM CLEMATIS	1 OZ OF WATER 5 DROPS 5 DROPS 3 DROPS 5 DROPS 7 SUCCUSSIONS	7 DROPS 5 TIMES
FLU	CLEMATIS STAR OF BETHLEHEM	1 OZ OF WATER 4 DROPS OF EACH FLOWER ESSENCE	ACUTE: 4 DROPS EVERY ½ HOUR
FLU	RESCUE REMEDY	5 DROPS	EVERY 5 MINUTES
FRAILTY	WILLOW	1 OZ OF WATER	3 DROPS

(PHYSICAL)		5 DROPS 30 SUCCUSSIONS	3 TIMES PER DAY FOR 2 WEEKS
FRAILTY (PHYSICAL)	MUSTARD OAK	1 OZ OF WATER 4 DROPS OF EACH FLOWER ESSENCE	4 DROPS 2 TIMES PER DAY FOR 5 DAYS
FRAILTY	MUSTARD OAK OLIVE	1 OZ OF WATER 4 DROPS OF EACH FLOWER ESSENCE	4 DROPS 2 TIMES PER DAY FOR 3 DAYS
GRIEF	CHERRY PLUM SCLERANTHUS RESCUE REMEDY	1 OZ OF WATER 5 DROPS 3 DROPS 11 DROPS	3 DROPS 5 TIMES PER DAY FOR 23 DAYS
GRIEF	OLIVE GORSE RESCUE REMEDY MUSTARD	2 OZ OF WATER 10 DROPS OF EACH FLOWER ESSENCE	5 DROPS AS NEEDED
GROUNDING	WILD OAT	FROM THE STOCK BOTTLE	4 DROPS 3 TIMES PER DAY FOR 3 DAYS
HALLUCINATION	CHERRY PLUM CLEMATIS AGRIMONY ROCK ROSE VERVAIN MIMULUS	FROM THE STOCK BOTTLE	4 DROPS OF EACH F/E 7 TIMES PER DAY FOR 3 WEEKS
INCONTINENCE	GORSE	1 OZ OF WATER	3 DROPS

	WILD OAT RESCUE REMEDY	3 DROPS OF EACH FLOWER ESSENCE	3 TIMES PER DAY FOR 5 DAYS
ITCH	RESCUE REMEDY	1 OZ OF WATER 4 DROPS OF F/E 7 SUCCUSSIONS	4 DROPS AS AS NEEDED
LIVER	LARCH ROCK ROSE WALNUT	1 OZ OF WATER 3 DROPS OF EACH FLOWER ESSENCE 24 SUCCUSSIONS	3 DROPS 2 TIMES PER DAY FOR 14 DAYS
MENTAL IMBALANCE	CHICORY CLEMATIS MUSTARD ROCK WATER WHITE CHESTNUT WILD OAT	1 OZ OF WATER 4 DROPS OF EACH FLOWER ESSENCE 45 SUCCUSSIONS	4 DROPS 2 TIMES PER DAY FOR 3 DAYS
MENTAL IMBALANCE	RESCUE REMEDY WILD ROSE IMPATIENS LARCH	1 OZ OF WATER 4 DROPS OF EACH FLOWER ESSENCES	5 DROPS 2 TIMES PER DAY FOR 6 DAYS
MENTAL IMBALANCE	AGRIMONY GORSE ROCK ROSE		5 DROPS OF EACH F/E 3 TIMES PER DAY FOR 9 DAYS
MENTAL IMBALANCE	ROCK WATER AGRIMONY	1 OZ OF WATER 5 DROPS OF EACH FLOWER ESSENCE	5 DROPS 4 TIMES PER DAY FOR 12 DAYS
MENTAL	AGRIMONY	1 OZ OF WATER	4 DROPS

EMOTIONAL IMBALANCE	BEECH MUSTARD RED CHESTNUT SCLERANTHUS WHITE CHESTNUT	4 DROPS OF EACH FLOWER ESSENCE	3 TIMES PER DAY FOR 7 DAYS
MENTAL EMOTIONAL IMBALANCE	RESCUE REMEDY IMPATIENS ROCK ROSE RED CHESTNUT	1 OZ OF WATER 5 DROPS OF EACH FLOWER ESSENCE 5 SUCCUSSIONS	4 DROPS 3 TIMES PER DAY FOR 5 DAYS
MENTAL EMOTIONAL IMBALANCE	GENTIAN GORSE HEATHER HOLLY RED CHESTNUT ROCK ROSE SCLERANTHUS	1 OZ OF WATER 5 DROPS OF EACH FLOWER ESSENCE	5 DROPS 2 TIMES PER DAY FOR 8 WEEKS
MENTAL EMOTIONAL OBSTACLES	IMPATIENS WILD OAT RESCUE REMEDY	1 OZ OF WATER 4 DROPS OF EACH FLOWER ESSENCE 65 SUCCUSSIONS	4 DROPS 2 TIMES PER DAY FOR 5 DAYS
MENTAL PHYSICAL IMBALANCE	SCLERANTHUS	1 OZ OF WATER 4 DROPS OF F/E	4 DROPS EVERY 15 MINUTES 6 TIMES
MENTAL SLUGGISHNESS	CHERRY PLUM MUSTARD	1 OZ OF WATER 4 DROPS OF EACH FLOWER ESSENCE 13 SUCCUSSIONS	3 DROPS EVERY ½ HOUR 4 TIMES, THEN EVERY HR. 5 TIMES
MUCOSA	RESCUE REMEDY	FROM THE STOCK	2 DROPS

(GUM)		BOTTLE	2 TIMES PER DAY FOR 15 DAYS
NAUSEA	RESCUE REMEDY CRAB APPLE	1 OZ OF WATER 4 DROPS OF EACH FLOWER ESSENCE	3 DROPS EVERY 5 MINUTES 6 TIMES
NERVE INJURY	RESCUE REMEDY	1 OZ OF WATER 8 DROPS OF EACH FLOWER ESSENCE	4 DROPS 4 TIMES PER DAY FOR 23 DAYS
NEUROSIS	CERATO MUSTARD ROCK WATER SCLERANTHUS STAR OF BETHLEHEM VERVAIN WALNUT WILD OAT	1 OZ OF WATER 5 DROPS OF EACH FLOWER ESSENCE	5 DROPS 5 TIMES PER DAY FOR 10 WEEKS
OSTEOARTHRITIS	CHICORY CLEMATIS	1 OZ OF WATER 4 DROPS OF EACH FLOWER ESSENCE	4 DROPS 2 TIMES PER DAY FOR 5 DAYS
PAIN	RESCUE REMEDY	FROM THE STOCK BOTTLE	3 DROPS EVERY 5 MINUTES 4 TIMES THEN 3 DROPS EVERY HOUR 8 TIMES
PAIN AND	CHICORY	1 OZ OF WATER	4 DROPS

STIFFNESS	GENTIAN RESCUE REMEDY	5 DROPS OF EACH FLOWER ESSENCE	3 TIMES PER DAY FOR 7 DAYS
PAIN (POST- OPERATIVE)	RESCUE REMEDY WILLOW	1 OZ OF WATER 4 DROPS OF EACH FLOWER ESSENCE	ACUTE: EVERY 5' 3 TIMES, THEN EVERY ½ HR 3 TIMES, THEN EVERY HR. UNTIL BETTER
PAIN (EMOTIONAL)	CHESTNUT BUD	FROM THE STOCK BOTTLE	2 DROPS 2 TIMES PER DAY FOR 5 DAYS
PARKINSON	ELM GENTIAN VERVAIN	1 OZ OF WATER 8 DROPS OF EACH FLOWER ESSENCE	4 DROPS 3 TIMES PER DAY FOR 5 DAYS
PARKINSON	HOLLY	1 OZ OF WATER 9 DROPS OF F/E 8 SUCCUSSIONS	5 DROPS 2 TIMES PER DAY FOR 1 DAY
PARKINSON	MIMULUS WILLOW	1 OZ OF WATER 4 DROPS OF EACH FLOWER ESSENCE	4 DROPS 2 TIMES PER DAY FOR 5 DAYS
PHYSICAL	STAR OF	1 OZ OF WATER	5 DROPS

IMBALANCE (GENERAL)	BETHLEHEM WHITE CHESTNUT WILD ROSE	12 DROPS OF EACH FLOWER ESSENCE	3 TIMES PER DAY FOR 5 DAYS
RHEUMATISM	HORNBEAM	1 OZ OF WATER 3 DROPS OF F/E	4 DROPS 2 TIMES PER DAY FOR 5 DAYS
RHEUMATISM	OAK ROCK ROSE SCLERANTHUS RESCUE REMEDY	1 OZ OF WATER 4 DROPS OF EACH FLOWER ESSENCE 75 SUCCUSSIONS	3 DROPS 3 TIMER PER DAY FOR 18 DAYS
ROSACEA	SCLERANTHUS RESCUE REMEDY	FROM THE STOCK BOTTLE	3 DROPS OF EACH F/E 3 TIMES PER DAY FOR 4 DAYS
SHOCK (POST)	WILLOW WILD OAT	FROM THE STOCK BOTTLE	4 DROPS OF EACH F/E 2 TIME PER DAY FOR 3 DAYS
SHOCK	SWEET CHESTNUT RESCUE REMEDY	1 OZ OF WATER 4 DROPS OF EACH FLOWER ESSENCE	3 DROPS 2 TIMES PER DAY FOR 4 DAYS
SIDE (RIGHT/ LEFT IMBALANCE)	ASPEN CHICORY CHESTNUT BUD	1 OZ OF WATER 7 DROPS 6 DROPS 7 DROPS	5 DROPS 2 TIMES PER DAY FOR 21 DAYS
STERILITY	CERATO	1 OZ OF WATER	3 DROPS

	CLEMATIS CRAB APPLE	5 DROPS OF EACH FLOWER ESSENCE 3 SUCCUSSIONS	2 TIMES PER DAY FOR 7 DAYS
STROKE (POST- CONVALECENCE)	HOLLY ROCK ROSE	1 OZ OF WATER 5 DROPS OF EACH FLOWER ESSENCE	5 DROPS 3 TIMES PER DAY FOR 7 DAYS
STROKE (POST)	SCLERANTHUS	1 OZ OF WATER 5 DROPS OF F/E 30 SUCCUSSIONS	5 DROPS 3 TIMES PER DAY FOR 4 DAYS
STROKE (POST) PREVENTION	CHICORY IMPATIENS LARCH OLIVE	1 OZ OF WATER 5 DROPS OF EACH FLOWER ESSENCE 10 SUCCUSSIONS	5 DROPS 2 TIMES PER DAY FOR 7 DAYS
STROKE (POST) PREVENTION	RESCUE REMEDY MUSTARD ASPEN PINE ROCK WATER SWEET CHESTNUT	1 OZ OF WATER 5 DROPS 5 DROPS 10 DROPS 10 DROPS 5 DROPS 5 DROPS 27 SUCCUSSIONS	9 DROPS 2 TIMES PER DAY FOR 4 MONTHS
TINNITUS	WILD OAT	FROM THE STOCK BOTTLE	3 DROPS 1 TIME
TINNITUS	AGRIMONY ASPEN ROCK ROSE	FROM THE STOCK BOTTLE	5 DROPS OF EACH F/E 1 TIME PER DAY FOR 14 DAYS
TOXIC	GORSE	FROM THE STOCK	3 DROPS

EMOTIONS	CRAB APPLE ASPEN WILD OAT GENTIAN	BOTTLE	OF EACH F/E 3 TIMES PER DAY FOR 4 WEEKS
TOXIC EMOTIONS	WATER VIOLET	FROM THE STOCK BOTTLE	4 DROPS 2 TIMES PER DAY FOR 4 DAYS
TREMORS	HORNBEAM WILLOW RESCUE REMEDY	1 OZ OF WATER 4 DROPS OF EACH FLOWER ESSENCE	3 DROPS 3 TIMES PER DAY FOR 6 DAYS
TOOTH (ABSCESS)	WHITE CHESTNUT AGRIMONY	FROM THE STOCK BOTTLE	6 DROPS OF EACH F/E 3 TIMES PER DAY FOR 6 DAYS
TRAUMAS (PAST)	HOLLY GORSE	FROM THE STOCK BOTTLE	1 DROP OF EACH F/E ON A BAND- AID. WEAR IT FOR 2 DAYS
URINARY INFECTION	OLIVE SCLERANTHUS STAR OF BETHLEHEM RESCUE REMEDY	1 OZ OF WATER 6 DROPS OF EACH FLOWER ESSENCE	3 DROPS 2 TIMES PER DAY FOR 17 DAYS
VERICOSE	AGRIMONY	1 OZ OF WATER	3 DROPS

VEINS	BEECH ELM	4 DROPS OF EACH FLOWER ESSENCE	2 TIMES PER DAY FOR 9 DAYS
VERTIGO	ASPEN CLEMATIS SCLERANTHUS	1 OZ OF WATER 6 DROPS OF EACH FLOWER ESSENCE 17 SUCCUSSIONS	4 DROPS 2 TIMES PER DAY FOR 7 DAYS
VISION (POOR)	WILLOW	FROM THE STOCK BOTTLE	3 DROPS 3 TIMES PER DAY FOR 4 WEEKS
VITALITY (GENERAL)	RESCUE REMEDY	1OZ OF WATER 4 DROPS OF F/E	3 DROPS 3 TIMES PER DAY FOR 6 DAYS
WALKING IMBALANCE	WILLOW	1 OZ OF WATER 5 DROPS OF F/E	5 DROPS 2 TIMES PER DAY FOR 3 WEEKS
WOUND HEALING	MUSTARD MIMULUS	1 OZ OF WATER 5 DROPS OF EACH 27 SUCCUSSIONS	5 DROPS 3 TIMES PER DAY FOR 2 DAYS
WOUND HEALING	CHESTNUT BUD WHITE CHESTNUT RESCUE REMEDY	1 OZ OF WATER 4 DROPS OF EACH 13 SUCCUSSIONS	SPRAY ON WOUND 3 TIMES PER DAY FOR 2 DAYS

DR.BACH
FLOWER ESSENCES'S
VIBRATIONAL CODES

"It is important that remedies chosen should be life-giving and uplifting; of such vibrations that elevate…" Dr. Edward Bach

DR. BACH'S FLOWER ESSENCES
VIBRATIONAL CODE *

The following codes have been identified by the author via radiesthetic testing. The vibratory range is from the lowest: 000, to the highest: 999.

COMMON NAME	SCIENTIFIC NAME	CODE
1. AGRIMONY	AGRIMONIA EUPHATORIA	690
2. ASPEN	POPULUS TREMULA	926
3. BEECH	FAGUS SYLVATICA	811
4. CENTAURY	CENTAURIUM UMBELLATUM	648
5. CERATO	CERATOSTIGMA WILLMOTTIANA	420
6. CHERRY PLUM	PRUNUS CERASIFERA	989
7. CHESTNUT BUD	AESCULUS HIPPOCASTANUM	888
8. CHICORY	CIHORIUM INTYBUS	375
9. CLEMATIS	CLEMATIS VITALBA	999

10. CRAB APPLE	MALUS PUMILA	666
11. ELM	ULMUS PROCERA	464
12. GENTIAN	GENTIANA AMARELLA	788
13. GORSE	ULEX EUROPOEUS	879
14. HEATHER	CALLUNA VULGARIS	333
15. HOLLY	ILEX AQUIFOLUM	706
16. HONEYSUCKLE	LONICERA CAPRIFOLIUM	374
17. HORNBEAM	CARPINUS BETULUS	704
18. IMPATIENS	IMPATIENS GLANDULIFERA	671
19. LARCH	LARIX DECIDUA	604
20. MIMULUS	MIMULUS GUTTATUS	550
21. MUSTARD	SINAPIS ARVENSIS	990
22. OAK	QUERCUS ROBUR	501
23. OLIVE	OLEA EUROPEA	607
24. PINE	PINUS SYLVESTRIS	438
25. RED CHESTNUT	AESCULUS CARNEA	866
26. ROCK ROSE	HELIANTHEMUM NUMMULARIUM	693
27. ROCK WATER		326
28. SCLERANTHUS	SCLERANTHUS ANNUUS	333
29. STAR OF BETHLEHEM	ORNITHOGALUM UMBELLATUM	435

30. SWEET CHESTNUT	CASTANEA SATIVA	341
31. VERVAIN	VERBENA OFFICIONALIS	441
32. VINE	VITIS VINIFERA	873
33. WALNUT	JUGLANS REGIA	473
34. WATER VIOLET	HOTTONIA PALUSTRIS	395
35. WHITE CHESTNUT	AESCULUS HIPPOCASTANUM	315
36. WILD OAT	BROMUS RAMOSUS	364
37. WILD ROSE	ROSA CANINA	424
38. WILLOW	SALIX VITELLINA	756
39. RESCUE REMEDY		999

CLOSING STATEMENT

" We must develop our personality and free ourselves from all worldly influences, obeying only the dictates of our soul." Dr. Edward Bach

CLOSING STATEMENT

During his address given at Southport, on February of 1931, entitled " You Suffer From Yourselves", Dr. Edward Bach made the following statement regarding his work:

" This is the natural continuation of Hahnemann's great work; the consequence of that line of thought which was disclosed to him, leading as a step further towards perfect understanding of disease and health, and is the stage to bridge the gap between where he left us and the dawn of that day when humanity will have reach that state of advancement when it can receive direct the glory of Divine healing".

The author of this book trusts that she has earned the temporary appropriation of the above statement and the addition of Dr. Bach's name next to Dr. Hanemann's, thus bridging " the gap between where they left us" and bringing us closer to the state of receiving " direct the glory of Divine healing".

BIBLIOGRAPHY

" *These remedies have the power to elevate vibrations and thus draw down spiritual power, which cleanses mind and body and heals.*"
Dr. Edward Bach

BIBLIOGRAPHY

1. Aurive, Marc. "Curso Practico de Radiestesia", 1995, Tikal, Spain.
2. Allen, H.C., Dr. " The Materia Medica of the Nosodes". B.Jain Publishers, New Delhi, India, 2004.
3. " Bach Flower Essences for the Family", 1999, Wigmore Publications, London, England.
4. Back, Dr., Edward. "Heal Thyself", 1931. The C.W. Daniel Co, 1996, England.
5. The Dr. Edward Bach Centre. " The Bach Flower Remedies", 1997. Keats Publishing, Inc. England.
6. Bach, Dr, Edward. " The Essential Writings of Edward Bach". Vermilion, London, 2005.
7. Ball, Stefan and Howard, Judy. "Emotional Healing for Cats", 2000. The C.W. Daniel Company Limited, England.
8. Ball, Stefan and Howard, Judy. " Bach flower Remedies for Animals", 1999. Vermilion, London, England.
9. Barnard, Julian, Editor. " Collected Writings of Edward Bach", 1987. Ashgrove Publishing, England.
10. Bear, N.D., Jessica. "Practical Uses and Applications of the Bach Flower Emotional Remedies", 1990. Balancing Essential Press.
11. Bhattacharyya, B, Dr. "Magnet Dowsing or Magnet Study of Life", 1992. Firma KLM Private Limited, Calcutta, India.

12. Blome, M.D., Gotz. " Advanced Bach Flower Therapy", 1999. Healing Arts Press, Rochester Vermont, USA.

13. Craydon, C.F.E.P., Deborah and Bellows, Lic.Ac., Warren. " Floral Acupuncture", 2005. The Crossing Press, Berkeley, Ca, USA.

14. Eden, Donna. " Energy Medicine", 1998. Penguin Putnam Inc. New York, USA.

15. De Hersaint, Jean-Pol. " Tout Par La Radiesthesie", 1973. Editions Dangles, Paris, France.

16. Gerula, Rev., Ricardo Luis. " Radiestesia Integral", 2005. Editorial Kier, S.A., Argentina.

17. Ghatak, Dr. N. " Chronic Disease-Its Cause and Cure", 1931. India.

18. Graham, Helen and Vlamis, Gregory. " Bach Flower Remedies for Animals". 1999. Findhorn Press, Scotland.

19. Gross, M.H. "Biorhythms", 1975. Herman Bauer Publishing Company. Germany.

20. Hahnemann, Dr, Samuel, "Chronic Diseases- Their Peculiar Nature and Their Homeopathic Cure". B.Jain Publishers, New Delhi, India, 2001.

21. Hahnemann, Dr. Samuel, "The Chronic Diseases- Theoretical Part". B. Jain Publishers, New Dehli, India, 2004.

22. Hasnas, M.S.W., Rachelle. " Pocket Guide to Bach Flower Essences", 1997. Freedom, California, USA.

23. Hasnas, M.S.W., Rachelle. "The Essence of Bach Flowers- Traditional and Transpersonal Use and Practice", 1999. The Crossing Press Freedom, California, USA.

24. Howard, Judy and Ramsell, John. " The Original Writings of Edward Bach", 1990. The C.W. Daniel Company Limited, England.

25. Julian, O.A., Dr. "Materia Medica of Nosodes with Repertory" B. Jain Publishers, New Delhi, India, 2000.

26. Kramer, Dietmar. "New Back Flower Body Maps", 1996. Healing Arts Press, Rochester, Vermont, USA.

27. Mathur, Dr., K.N. " Principles of Prescribing", 2006. B. Jain Publishers, Ltd. India

28. Moine, Michel. " La Radiestesia", 1973. Editions Stock, Spain.

29. Motura, M.D., Giraldo Nestor. " Learn to Cure Yourself with Flower Essences and Homeopathy", 7th edition, 1999. Lux Printing S.A., Santa Fe, Argentina.

30. Motura, M.D., Giraldo Nestor. " Aprende a Curarte", 24th edition, 2005. Fundacion Apis, Santa Fe Argentina.

31. Olson, Dale, W. " The Pendulum Charts- Knowing Your Intuitive Mind". 2005. Crystalline Publications, Eugene, Oregon, USA.

32. O'Neil, Barbara and Phillips, Richard. " Biorhythms- How to Live With Your Life Cycles", 1975. Ward Ritchie Press, Pasadena, California, USA.

33. Ortega, Proceso Sanchez, Dr. "Notes on the Miasms or Hahnemann's Chronic Diseases". Published by the Homeopathic Pharmacy, New Delhi, India, 1980.

34. Scheffer, Mechthild. " Bach Flower Therapy", 1987. Thorsons Publisher, Rochester, Vermont, USA.

35. Weeks, Nora. " Medical Discoveries of Edward Bach, Physician", 1973. New Canaan, Ct, Keats Publishing Co. England.

36. Wheeler, Dr, F.J. " The Bach Remedies Repertory", 1952. Saffron Walden, The C.W. Daniel Company Limited, England,

37. Weeks, Nora and Bullen, Victor. " The Bach Flower Remedies", 1964. Saffron Walden. The C.W. Daniel Company Limited, England.

LaVergne, TN USA
28 November 2010
206557LV00004B/67/P

9 781593 306458